Final MB

to Gillian, James, Richard and Hugh

For Churchill Livingstone:

Publisher: Laurence Hunter
Project Editor: Janice Urquhart
  Copy Editor: Adam Campbell
Project Controller: Nancy Arnott
Design Direction: Erik Bigland

Final MB

A Guide to Success in Clinical Medicine

H. R. Dalton BSc DPhil MRCP DipMedEd

With a contribution by
N. J. Reynolds BSc MD MRCP

Foreword by
K. B. Saunders
Professor of Medicine, St George's Hospital Medical School, London

SECOND EDITION

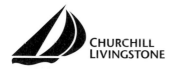

CHURCHILL LIVINGSTONE

NEW YORK EDINBURGH LONDON MADRID MELBOURNE SAN FRANCISCO
AND TOKYO 1997

CHURCHILL LIVINGSTONE
Medical Division of Pearson Professional Limited

Distributed in the United States of America by Churchill
Livingstone Inc., 650 Avenue of the Americas, New York,
N.Y. 10011, and by associated companies, branches and
representatives throughout the world.

First edition 1991
Second edition 1997

ISBN 0 443 05332 4

British Library Cataloguing in Publication Data
A catalogue record for this book is available from the British
Library

Library of Congress Cataloging in Publication Data
A catalog record for this book is available from the Library of
Congress

Medical knowledge is constantly changing. As new
information becomes available, changes in treatment,
procedures, equipment and the use of drugs become
necessary. The author and the publishers have, as far as it is
possible, taken care to ensure that the information given in
the text is accurate and up to date. However, readers are
strongly advised to confirm that the information, especially
with regard to drug usage, complies with current legislation
and standards of practice.

The
publisher's
policy is to use
**paper manufactured
from sustainable forests**

Printed by Longman Singapore Publishers (Pte) Ltd

Contents

Foreword

Passing finals is a question of doing simple things well. The process is mainly designed to detect the small percentage of students who are not ready to perform as house physicians or surgeons, so that they can be given further undergraduate training (and also to detect a small proportion of high-fliers). The ambition of any Dean or Professor of Medicine is to get a 100% pass rate, but they are almost always frustrated. This gives no pleasure: it is no fun failing students and examining resits is a terrible bore.

If you are a passenger in a motor car, you can usually tell within a few minutes whether the driver is competent or not, though it would often be difficult to say precisely how. When an examiner watches a student examining an abdomen or using an ophthalmoscope, it is usually rapidly obvious whether the student is competent, regardless of their findings. You can 'miss the spleen' and still pass. Techniques of clinical examination need practising until they become automatic: when they do, and if they are done right, the practitioner looks competent.

There are, however, certain tricks of the trade handed down from generation to generation, which are worth knowing. They involve obvious things like dress, but also more subtle matters. These are well set out by Dr Dalton. There is also, whether examiners like it or not, a corpus of experience in the practical clinical field outside which the examination can rarely stray. You will see mitral stenosis, possibly for the first time. You won't see hypoglycaemic coma. Finally, there are questions or topics which come up frequently and are worth special revision.

Don't confuse this book with a textbook of medicine. Do use it as you would use revision ward rounds in the months before finals. Dr Dalton is a highly regarded teacher and what he writes makes good sense. I don't agree with all of it, but then, I often passed students who said things I didn't agree with, provided such points weren't too numerous, and were well argued.

London   K. B. S.

Preface

This book is intended primarily for final year medical students who are preparing for their final clinical examination in General Medicine. It is not written as a complete textbook of medicine and should not be treated as such. It is very much an exam-orientated book, and is meant to alleviate some of the suffering of those nail-biting weeks just prior to the final MB. It concentrates on the type of questions asked by the examiners and how to respond in a way which will give the candidate the best chance of success. The majority of the book concentrates on the short cases, as from my experience students find these the most difficult. I have also included sections on the written paper, the long cases and the viva.

At the end of some of the chapters there is a 'key questions' section. This consists of some questions which are amongst the more frequently asked, and are included for you to consider. You will find many, but not all, of the answers in the main text. If you can't find the answer discuss it with your colleagues, or look it up in one of those big fat reference books.

Cornwall 1996   H. R. D.

Acknowledgements

I would like to thank the following for their help with the second edition: Mr Teifi James, Dr Nick Reynolds, Dr David Gould, Dr Rod Harvey, Chris Lloyd, Isabel Flemons.

Cornwall 1996   H. R. D.

PART 1

GENERAL PRINCIPLES

1.1

The examination

The final MB examination varies among different medical schools. However, in general terms, there is always a written section and a clinical section.

THE WRITTEN PAPER

Past papers are available and it is essential to get hold of these to see what you are up against. 'Question spotting' is notoriously inaccurate and not to be recommended, but practising your answering technique in both the multiple choice questions (MCQs) and essay section is definitely worthwhile. I would suggest that you ask one of your tutors (preferably someone who marks the real thing) to go over your model answers with you.

Most MCQs in medicine are marked in a sophisticated manner these days. The following scheme is widely used:

- correct response = + 1
- incorrect response = − 1
- no response = 0.

In addition to this, questions are often graded as to the degree of difficulty, so that a correct answer to a difficult question carries relatively more weight than to an easy one. The trick is to try and answer the right number of questions (approximately 85–90% of the total), avoid wild guesses and try to avoid answering easy questions incorrectly. Admittedly this is easier said than done, but attempting past papers will help you gain more confidence. The written section is generally 'close-marked' and so to miss out a question completely can be totally disastrous. Having said this, if it happens to you, don't start sharpening up the bread knife! I have known several people do this and still pass. You must practise your examination technique on the essay questions and pay particular attention to:

- Time allocation to each answer.
- Structure of the answer. Make it easier for the examiner to read and mark by setting it out in clearly headed sections.
- Legibility. It has been shown in several studies that answers written in good legible script gain better marks. You need to balance this against allocation of time.
- Answering a question you know nothing about. You may not realise it but there will be relatively few things you know absolutely nothing about. Most questions, you should, at least, have some vague idea about. I recommend leaving the question you know least about until last. Doing good answers to the other questions you know more about will give you confidence and a chance to mull over the grey area of your last question at the back of your mind.

When you come to put pen to paper for the final question, you may realise you know more about it than you at first thought. If you are still having trouble you could put the subject matter of the question through a 'sieve' and see what comes out at the other end. There are many such 'sieves' in local usage — I recommend my students make up their own, as these mnemonics are more easily remembered. However, an example of such a 'sieve' is as follows (TIN CAN BEDD):

Trauma **I**nfection **N**eoplasia
Congenital **A**utoimmune **N**utritional
Blood (i.e. haematological) **E**ndocrine **D**rugs **D**octors

Whatever you do, put *something* down on paper as your answer to that difficult question. A blank sheet will score 0 out of 10; a dreadful answer may score 3 out of 10. This is an enormous difference in a close-marked paper.

I will say no more about the written paper. Obviously it is essential to do the necessary book-work to pass, but I think attention to the above points will help a little knowledge go further.

THE CLINICAL PAPER

The clinical section directly involves patients and is divided into two sections: 'long case' and the 'short cases'. The clinical section is usually held in a purpose-built room, which comprises a number of clinical cubicles and some cubicles for the examiners. The cases can be drawn from all specialities of medicine. Some medical schools (but not all) include psychiatric and paediatric cases in the clinical paper.

The long case

Candidates are usually given 45 minutes to take a history from and examine a long case. However, in some centres students are expected to take a psychiatric history and are therefore given 1 hour. In addition to this, 20 minutes are set aside for the candidates to explain the history and physical findings to the examiners. You may well be taken back to the patient to demonstrate the clinical signs which you have elicited. The long cases are discussed in more detail in Part 2.

The short cases

Thirty minutes are set aside for you to be examined on short cases. A pair of examiners will take you to a number of cases and ask you to perform a clinical examination under direct observation. Most students find this the most stressful part of the examination. The short cases are discussed in more detail in Part 3.

The viva

At the end of the examination there is the viva voce. This entails a 20 minute interview with two examiners. In the Final MB viva the examiners can be from any field of general medicine or the allied specialities of paediatrics, psychiatry, community medicine, dermatology, geriatrics, etc. The primary purpose of this exercise is to assess a candidate's clinical problem-solving ability, and questions are often posed as clinical scenarios. Having said this, the examiners are free to ask whatever type of question they like and frequently do so.

The viva is used to distinguish borderline (pass/fail) candidates and those who may be awarded a distinction. In some medical schools, therefore, only a proportion of candidates will be invited to attend the viva. In other centres all candidates will have a viva. The viva is discussed in more detail in Part 4.

1.2

Examiners and the candidate

THE EXAMINERS

The clinical examiners traditionally work in pairs. If the examination paper is an 'internal' one there will be one examiner from your teaching hospital group and one examiner who has been invited from outside. If the examination is 'external' both examiners will be alien to your previous experience.

You are usually told several days in advance who your examiners are and where they are from. It is helpful to find out a little about them, particularly if they have any 'foibles'. Some examiners have particular ways they like the abdomen examined, for example. If you know any students from the medical school at which the examiner works it is well worth a 10p phone call to find out such information in advance. Check with candidates from your own medical school from previous years, as they may have met them in the exam setting and could possibly give you valuable tips.

You must remember that the examiners may have to examine for 4 or 5 days. They are human (believe it or not) and are subject to feelings of hunger, boredom and irritability like the rest of us. This should not affect you in any serious way. However, if you are ever in the position of being the registrar who organises the examination, please make sure the mid-morning coffee and biscuits arrive on time, or you may find yourself looking for another job!

Individual medical school pass rates are, in general, remarkably constant from year to year. The reason for this is not hard to discern: if they were to fail 30% of candidates one year and only 10% of candidates the next year this would create havoc in the employment market place. One year there would not be enough newly qualified doctors to fill the available house physician/surgeon posts, the next year there would be a glut of new doctors with consequent medical unemployment. The first scenario would not be popular with our senior medical colleagues, who would be at sea without a houseman. The second would not be popular with Her Majesty's Government, who are uneasy about unemployment at the best of times.

Having said that, the pass rate varies little from year to year; there are occasional hiccups when considerably more students fail than in previous years. The reasons for this are not entirely clear. It seems difficult to believe that the overall standard of candidate would vary much from year to year, especially in schools which have over 100 students per year. It is possible that the reasons for such discrepancies lie with the 'rogue examiner' who insists on failing more candidates than usual. Such examiners could be external ('these X students are useless compared to my Y students') or internal (e.g. a new head of department wanting either to stamp his authority on his new medical school or to teach the students a lesson they will not forget 'for not turning up to my teaching sessions').

THE CANDIDATE: WHAT THE EXAMINERS ARE LOOKING FOR

In the final MB examination the examiners are trying to pass you (as opposed to trying to fail you, which is the situation in most postgraduate examinations). The attributes which the examiners are looking for are those which make a good house doctor and they can be summarised by the 'three Cs':

* competence (and common sense)
* caring
* conventionality.

Any serious deviation from these three attributes would result in the candidate being invited to reattend in 6 months' time.

Competence

The candidate must create the impression that she is used to being with patients; that she can do a quick, thorough examination (which looks professional); and that she can talk in common sense terms about her findings.

Caring

The candidate must demonstrate a caring attitude to his patients during the examination. Never hurt the patient. *Always* ask the patient if he is comfortable. Introduce yourself to the patient at the start, and ask permission to examine the relevant part or parts. You will be under intense stress during the examination, but remember that the patient has feelings too; *never* put the patient in an embarrassing position.

Conventionality

You must appear to be conventional, even if you are not. Men should wear a conventional suit in blue or grey, white shirt, plain tie and black shoes. Hair should be short but conservative. Women should wear a smart dress or a two piece — nothing too revealing or outrageous. Attitudes should be conventional. Always call patients by their name: Mr X or Mrs Y. Try to smile and be confident. Do not be overconfident. Examiners do not like this, and with good reasons. Do not try to tell jokes or be too jovial.

On no account must you argue with the examiner — even if you know you are right. Examiners regard this as insulting. More importantly, they will probably fail you. Such overconfidence is considered in a poor light. The reason for this is that when housemen are overconfident and unaware of their personal professional limitations they seriously jeopardise the health of their patients: this may cause unnecessary suffering and possibly death. Examiners, therefore, often fail overconfident candidates, and this usually comes as a nasty shock to the person involved.

In summary, you have to give the examiner the impression that, if his mother were ill, he would not mind you being the doctor looking after her.

1.3

Equipment

MIND AND BODY

The most important piece of equipment is yourself: your mind and body must be sharp and in good working order on the big day. It is up to you to make sure that this is the case. Do not stay up all night before the day of the examination learning the 25 causes of atrial fibrillation, as you will be in no fit state to remember them in the high-pressure setting of the examination room. Get an early night if you can. A tot of whisky may help you sleep. I do not recommend any other kind of hypnotic.

A few candidates go to extreme lengths during the run-up to the examinations. Some stay up all night trying to cram in those extra facts, filling themselves with endless cups of strong coffee. This is not recommended. Try to appreciate the difference between the time spent revising when you are alert and when you are not. A good hour's work when your mind is sharp is worth at least three when you are overtired with caffeine toxicity.

One or two candidates get so wound up by feelings of impending doom that they resort to pharmacological manipulations to try to improve their performance during the revision period, or the examination itself. I cannot stress how important it is to avoid this. It is a recipe for disaster. If you are in this position you ought to go and see someone you trust (preferably a doctor), *now*. Drugs which have been used are caffeine-based stimulants (to keep awake to revise), hypnotics (to sleep after a hard day's revising) and beta-blockers (to keep calm).

All of the above drugs have central nervous system effects and will impair your mental agility on the day. Do not take them. A couple of drinks at 10.30 p.m. in the local pub with colleagues after a hard day's revision is much kinder on the central nervous system, and infinitely more pleasant.

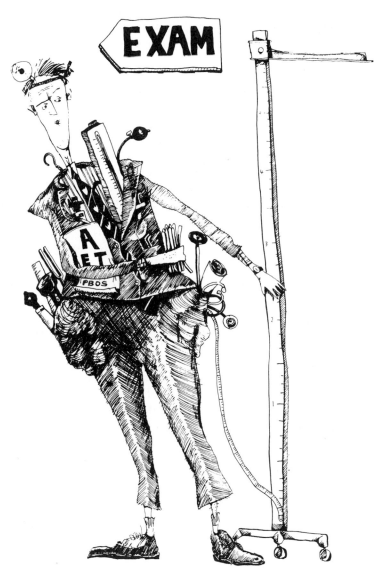

'Oh dear, I think I've forgotten my cotton wool balls.'

EQUIPMENT TO TAKE WITH YOU

Stethoscope

You should take your own stethoscope with you. This should be an ordinary one. If you bring out a £200 Littman Cardiology or St George's device the examiners may expect you to be able to hear the really difficult murmurs. This is called asking for trouble.

You need to check that it works properly before the exam. A contemporary of mine had the earpieces of his stethoscope blocked up as a practical joke (by so-called 'friends') prior to his clinical finals! He could not hear a thing through it during the exam, but luckily he still managed to pass.

Ophthalmoscope

You ought to take your own, for several reasons. If you have not got one don't worry — one will be provided. Ophthalmoscopes vary in design; it is important to get to know yours before the exam. Get to know which knobs do what, and make sure the batteries are new and the lenses are clean.

Neurological equipment

This will be provided at the examination. It is probably worth having some simple sensory testing equipment such as:

• *throw away* pins (HIV risk)
• cotton wool ball
• tape measure.

These will not take up much room in your pockets.

Tuning forks, patella hammers, smell bottles, Snellen charts, etc. are best left for the medical school to provide, as they are rather bulky items.

PART 2

THE LONG CASE

2

The long case

THE LONG CASE

Candidates are usually given 45 minutes to take a history from and examine a long case. However, in some centres students are expected to take a psychiatric history and are therefore given 1 hour. In addition to this, 20 minutes are set aside for the candidate to explain the history and physical findings to the examiners. You may well be taken back to the patient to demonstrate the clinical signs that you have elicited.

In any examination setting, assessment of students is made in three broad areas:

- knowledge
- attitudes
- skills.

In the long case all three of these areas will be assessed. You will need to demonstrate a sound knowledge of basic medical principles. The examiners will also be looking for you to demonstrate a professional attitude towards both themselves and the patient. However, the most important area under scrutiny is the area of clinical skills, and in particular communication skills. By this I mean the ability to take a history from a patient, integrate this with your findings on clinical examination and then communicate this succinctly to the examiners. This does not mean that clinical examination skills are not tested in the long case (they certainly are), but it is not the primary purpose of this part of the examination. This contrasts sharply with the short cases where the main purpose is to assess your ability at clinical examination.

Patients

The patients for the long case may be taken from the disciplines of general medicine, geriatric medicine, psychiatry or paediatrics. They are usually selected for the examination because of their ability to give a clear history. Occasionally a candidate may get a patient who, for one reason or another, cannot give a clear history. This may cause you to panic — but don't. Simply do the best you can under the conditions and explain to the examiners that you had difficulty taking a reliable history and the reasons for it. For example, the patient could be demented, have a malfunctioning hearing aid, or be dysarthric or unable to speak English. You might like to suggest to the examiners that you would like to demonstrate why the history was so difficult to obtain (they may not have realised this). This would involve, for example, doing an abbreviated mental test score on the patient, or the demonstration of dysarthria in a patient with a cerebellar syndrome. Try to build up a rapport with the patient — she may tell you what the diagnosis is. The 'professional patient' (i.e. one who is frequently called up for examinations) may even know what clinical signs she is supposed to have!

The patients are drawn from two sources. Firstly, there are the in-patients. These are patients who have been admitted as an emergency to hospital in the days prior to the examination. They will be in the recovery phase from their current illness. Very sick patients should never be included in the examination. Current in-patients tend to be in a minority. This is simply a matter of logistics for the people organising the examination. There are usually not enough patients who are fit enough, able to give a good history, or have interesting clinical signs to go round.

The numbers are made up from out-patients who are brought in specially for the examination. These are people with (usually) chronic physical signs, who can give a good history. Most centres have a list of patients on whom they call, which is added to and subtracted from each year. Among their number will be 'professional patients' who have been used numerous times before. They are often the most helpful to candidates, for reasons already outlined.

Paediatric cases can be daunting. Trying to get a history from and examine an uncooperative child can be a nightmare. You *must* get the parent(s) on your side. They are usually very well informed about the condition their child is suffering from. Enlist the parent's help in both the history and examination as much as possible. If all else fails you can always ask the parent what the diagnosis is and what treatment the patient is having — she may also know what the physical signs are.

Psychiatric cases are usually straightforward. You will know if you have a psychiatric long case because the registrar will usually tell you that a 'physical examination is unnecessary'. The case will either be depressed, manic or schizophrenic. Occasional cases of anorexia, bulimia, alcohol-related problems, obsessive/compulsive behaviour or personality disorder are included.

The long case history

It is important to ask the patient's name. I have heard of a candidate who went to see a long case and could find absolutely nothing wrong in the history or examination. He told the examiners this, and they duly took him back to the patient:

Examiner (to the patient):   'What is your name, sir?'
Patient: 'Napoleon Bonaparte.'

The history should be written down on paper as it is taken. Paper is provided. This should be done in the formalised traditional method which you have been taught since your first day on the wards (see Table 2.1). The examiners are very keen on the social history — in other words how the patient's illness affects his/her daily life. You should find out all the details regarding Meals on Wheels, home helps, district nurse, social worker, steps at home, Zimmer frames, sticks, crutches, getting out of the house, day centres, which room the patient sleeps in, family, neighbours, care-givers, GP home visits, financial problems, etc., etc.

Table 2.1
Name:
Age:
Occupation:
Main complaint:
History of present complaint:
Past medical history:
Current medication:
Known allergies:
Family history:
Social history:
Systems review:

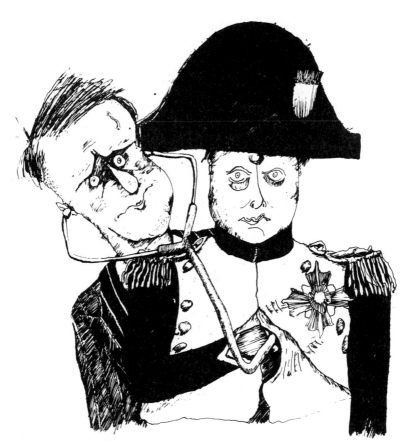

'Not tonight, Josephine.'

Examining the long case

You must perform a quick, but thorough, examination. You must, obviously, pay particular attention to the relevant areas indicated by your history: do not miss *anything* out. A generalised scheme for examination is set out in Table 2.2.

There is a lot to get through in the time allocated. A detailed neurological examination must be done, but clearly if time is a problem and no neurological pathology is indicated by the history, it may be necessary to curtail this to a brief version. It is most important *not* to examine the genitalia or perform a PR examination, but it is essential to express the desire to do so. Do not forget to take the blood pressure, look in the sputum pot and look for clues

Table 2.2

General observation
Breasts
Thyroid
Skin
Evidence of jaundice, anaemia, cyanosis, clubbing, lymphadenopathy
Scars

Cardiovascular system
Pulse, blood pressure, JVP
Apex beat, heart sounds 1 and 2, additional sounds, murmurs
Thrill, heaves, palpable heart sounds
Peripheral pulses, peripheral oedema
Bruits
Retinae

Respiratory system
Respiratory rate (breaths per minute)
Trachea
Chest expansion
Percussion note
Breath sounds
Tactile vocal fremitus, auditory resonance, whispering pectoriloquy
Sputum pot

Abdomen
General observation: observation of abdomen for obvious fullness, mass or scars
Signs of chronic liver disease
Tenderness, rebound?, guarding?
Masses
Organs: liver, kidneys, spleen, bladder, gravid uterus
Hernial orifices
Percussion
Bowel sounds

Central nervous system
Orientation
• time   • person
• place
Cranial nerves I–XII
Tone
Power
Reflexes
Sensation
• light touch   • joint position sense
• pain   • vibration sense
Gait
Cerebellar signs
Jaw jerk, Romberg's sign

left by the examiners, for example, temperature and peak flow charts or diabetic drinks on the locker. If there is a sample of the patient's urine, test it. If there is no urine testing kit ask for it, or tell the examiners that none was available.

Presenting the long case

Forty-five minutes may not seem a long time but, with practice under examination conditions, it is usually more than adequate. It is best to try to finish the case within 40 minutes, so leaving a valuable 5 minutes thinking time. This will give you a chance to gather your thoughts, and it will also give you an opportunity to decide which aspect of the case to bring out when you present the case to the examiners. I strongly recommend you use this time to summarise the case in *writing*. You should always write down the history and examination in any case, as it is often helpful, and sometimes necessary, to refer to your notes during your presentation. At the end I recommend that you write five brief paragraphs (of two to three sentences each) in summary:

- summary of the history
- summary of the clinical findings
- differential diagnosis
- investigations you think necessary
- relevant treatment — both immediate and long-term.

When you come to present your findings you must do so in a thorough and methodical manner. This means going through all the aspects of the history and examination in turn. It is important to emphasise the positive findings and relevant negative findings in the light of your final diagnosis. This prevents the presentation becoming a 10-minute monotone. At the end of the presentation offer a brief summary of the case together with a diagnosis or differential diagnosis.

The examiners expect candidates to give a concise, thorough and intelligent account of the case they have seen, presented in a formal way. They will tell you if they want something else. After the presentation the examiner will ask questions such as:

- what is the differential diagnosis?
- how would you investigate this patient?
- what do you think of this patient's treatment?
- how would you have managed this patient in casualty?
- come and demonstrate the physical signs which you have elicited.

Occasionally, the examiners will stop you midway through your presentation, or even before you have got properly started and ask one of the above questions. This is a technique employed frequently by the media when interviewing politicians, and can be most disconcerting if you are not expecting it. If you have allowed yourself 5 minutes thinking time and made some notes before your presentation you will be better able to handle this more aggressive approach.

See as many long cases as you can to practise your technique. Present cases to each other, and to the houseman, registrar and consultant — in fact, anybody you can get to listen. Get them to criticise you constructively. Think about their criticisms.

Some people have great difficulty communicating verbally, particularly under stress. I recommend that if you are such a candidate you get a dictaphone and practise presenting the case to the machine. Play it back and listen to what you sound like. Remember that the machine does not lie. Keep on practising until you are perfect.

Tips

- Allow 5 minutes thinking time
- Summarise in writing
- Practise.

EXAMPLES OF LONG CASES

I have included two examples of common clinical problems which frequently crop up as long cases. The first one is a patient who is in the recovery phase from an uncomplicated myocardial infarction. The second case is an elderly woman who has been undergoing intensive rehabilitation in a geriatric ward after gradually becoming unable to manage at home. For each case I have set out the history and examination as you might write it down during your long case. After reading each case, try to write down the summary of the case, much as you would do during the final 5 minutes 'thinking' time at the end of your long case in the exam. Remember the summary headings are history, examination, differential diagnosis, investigations and management.

Case 1: The straightforward case

Name:	Mr J. S.
Age:	58 years
Occupation:	Salesman
c/o:	Chest pain
HPC:	Central crushing chest pain 6 days ago whilst watching TV. Radiated to left arm and jaw. Associated with nausea, vomiting and sweatiness. The patient's wife called the ambulance. The pain lasted 2 hours until he had an injection in casualty department. It was the worst pain he has ever had. He has had no episodes of chest pain before or since. No other associated symptoms.
PMH:	Nil
Drugs:	Nil
Allergies:	Nil
FH:	— mother died at age 80 from carcinoma of the breast — father has senile dementia and is in a nursing home 80 miles away — one brother only. He died of a myocardial infarction at the age of 53, 10 years ago.
SH:	Works as a salesman for a local company. Enjoys work but finds it demanding as it involves travel. Full and active social life. Happily married with 3 children (who are all well). Normal sex life. Drinks 30 units of alcohol per week (on average) and smokes 15 cigarettes per day (for 40 years). Finds driving to see his father twice a week stressful.
Systems review:	Normal
Clinical examination:	Normal

Summary of case 1

This is a 58-year-old previously fit salesman with a 2-hour history of cardiac chest pain relieved by an injection (of ? diamorphine). His risk factors for ischaemic heart disease include smoking and family history (brother).

Examination

The clinical examination was normal.

Diagnosis

The most likely diagnosis is that of an acute myocardial infarction, but the differential diagnosis includes:

- acute angina pectoris
- pericarditis
- oesophageal spasm
- musculoskeletal pain
- acute dissection of thoracic aorta.

Investigations

The following should be carried out:

- serial ECGs, cardiac enzymes and a CXR
- exercise ECG ⎫ as dictated by
- coronary angiography ⎭ subsequent symptoms

Acute management issues

Speed of arrival at hospital.   His wife was correct to call an ambulance straight away. Doing this for patients with an acute myocardial infarction will usually minimise delays before thrombolytic therapy can be administered and this improves prognosis.

Immediate diagnosis and treatment.   On arrival at hospital the patient should be rapidly assessed clinically and an ECG and CXR arranged. Pain relief (intravenous diamorphine) should be administered, if not already given, together with an anti-emetic. The patient should be given oral aspirin and intravenous streptokinase as soon as possible, based on the ECG evidence. The patient should be nursed on the coronary care unit.

Longer term management issues

- Use of ACE inhibitors in patients with anterior myocardial infarction or clinical signs of pulmonary oedema. This improves prognosis.
- Continued use of aspirin.
- Advise patient to stop smoking.
- Check lipid profile. Cholesterol may require lowering by diet and/or drugs.
- Cardiac rehabilitation programme. Stepped exercise care programme for patients post MI. Return to full activity after 6–8 weeks.
- Patients' concerns — future health, driving, work and sex life.

Case 2: The complex case — 'acopia'

Name:	Mrs P. D.
Age:	86 years
Occupation:	Retired school teacher
c/o:	Two weeks ago patient found on floor by her next-door neighbour.
HPC:	Mrs P. D. has had numerous falls at home over the last 6 months. She has become increasingly unsteady on her feet and has had some pain and reduced function of the right hip (which has been gradually getting worse) for the last 2 weeks. Thirty-six hours prior to her admission she tripped over a mat on the floor of her lounge and could not get up. She called out but could not make anyone hear. She stayed on the floor all night until her neighbour found her in the morning. She has been an in-patient since this time.
PMH:	Appendectomy 1936 Hysterectomy 1958 Cholecystectomy 1972 Hypertension since 1977 Ischaemic heart disease 1986 Atrial fibrillation 1992

Case 2 (*contd*)

Pulmonary oedema 1993
Admitted with acute confusional state 1994
due to? UTI

Drugs:
Digoxin, 0.125 mg od
Frumil T, od
Lisinopril, 5 mg od
Atenolol, 50 mg od
Quinine sulphate, 300 mg nocte
Temazepam, 10 mg nocte

Allergies:
Nil

FH:
— parents unknown (orphan)
— no children or brothers and sisters.

SH:
The patient has lived in the same house for 50 years. She worked as a primary school teacher at the local school for 35 years until her retirement at the age of 65. She is a well known figure in the local community, but has been unable to go out alone since the death of her husband 3 years ago. Over the last 2 years she has not been out at all. She is fiercely independent and has managed to cook all her own meals. Her main source of social support is her next-door neighbour who does her shopping, fetches her pension and tidies the house for her.

The patient's house is a bungalow, with two bedrooms (ground floor). She is connected to mains electricity and water, but not gas. She is on the telephone. There are six steps up to the front door and no handrail. The patient had been managing to get around the house by clutching onto furniture and using a walking stick.

Although Mrs P. D. has not been out of the house for 2 years she has several regular visitors to her house and maintains her interests in music and literature, although recently she has been having problems with her eyesight.

Case 2   (*contd*)

> She has refused meals on wheels in the past (she did not like them) and did have a home help, but she 'sacked' her because she did not tidy properly. The patient has no financial problems, and is a life-long teetotaller and non-smoker.

Systems

CVS: Hypertension since 1977. Well controlled. Has been on atenolol for 10 years. Patient has had occasional attacks of cardiac chest pain which last approximately 30 minutes and are relieved by GTN spray. She has not needed to use the spray for 18 months.

> Intermittent palpitations for 5 years associated with paroxysms of breathlessness. This has been much better since taking digoxin, frumil and lisonopril, although over the last few months she has been more breathless than usual, particularly in bed at night. Over the 2 months prior to admission her ankles were much more swollen.

RS, GIT: NAD

CNS: Main problem is deteriorating vision in both eyes. It is now difficult for the patient to read even large-print books using a magnifying glass.

M/S: Increasing pain and stiffness of the right hip for the last 2 years. She has had several falls in her house and she has had the hip X-rayed twice in the last 18 months.

Examination

— pleasant woman, lucid
— orientated in time, place and person
— mental test score 10/10
— no lymph nodes, jaundice, anaemia, clubbing or cyanosis.

Case 2   (*contd*)

CVS: p80 atrial fibrillation, BP 150/80, lying and
                    sitting
                    JVP raised 3 cm
                    AB displaced to mid-axillary line
                    HS I & II & III

Chest: Inspiratory crackles at both bases

Abdomen: Previous surgical scars, otherwise normal

CNS: Normal examination apart from bilateral
                    cataracts (fundoscopy impossible)

M/S: Tender on movement of right hip. Movement
                    limited to 40° flexion, 20° abduction. No
                    internal/external rotation possible.

Urine
analysis: Normal

**THIS WILL BE MORE DIFFICULT TO SUMMARISE
THAN CASE 1**

Summary of case 2

This is quite a complex case and to help you summarise succinctly
you need to identify the patient's problems and decide whether
they are active or inactive:

- active problems   — frequent falls
                       — poor eyesight
                       — breathlessness
                       — unable to get out of house
- inactive problems   — hypertension
                       — palpitations.

The next step is to 'SOAP' these active problems. This is a method
of problem analysis using the following scheme:

- **S**ubjective — the patient's complaint
- **O**bjective — relevant physical findings
- **A**ssessment — what you think the cause is
- **P**lan — what you intend to do about it.

Applying this approach to our case's active problems:

1. **S** — falls/poor mobility

   O — ? OA right hip, exclude old fracture, bilateral cataracts, takes temazepam

   A — falls due to a combination of OA of hip and poor eyesight due to cataracts. The layout/furniture of patient's house may be contributing. Patient is also taking temazepam which sometimes has a hangover effect causing inco-ordination in the elderly

   P — X-ray right hip. Discuss cataract surgery and refer if appropriate. Occupational therapy assessment including home visit. Stop temazepam.

2. **S** — poor eyesight

   O — bilateral cataracts

   A — cause is cataracts

   P — discuss cataract surgery and refer.

3. **S** — breathlessness

   O — signs of congestive cardiac failure. Patient takes a β-blocker

   A — atenolol may be contributing to the congestive cardiac failure

   P — stop atenolol. Monitor clinical response.

4. **S** — unable to get out of house

   O — as (1) and (2)

   A — as (1) and (2) but steps to front door may be contributing

   P — ask social services, occupational therapy to assess.

This seems rather a laborious process, but you are now in a position to summarise your findings in a succinct and rational way.

Summary

Mrs P. D. is an 86-year-old widow who was admitted to hospital 2 weeks ago after spending all night on the floor after a fall. She has had numerous falls recently and is finding it increasingly difficult to manage at home. Mrs P. D. has several active problems including poor mobility, poor eyesight, breathlessness and inability to get out of the house.

You can now use your problem list as a basis for further discussion.

PART 3

SHORT CASES

NB   Please note the following symbols which are used throughout this part
      of the book:

  * — indicates cases that frequently crop up in the final MB
  † — indicates more complicated cases that occur only rarely.

3.1

General approach

Thirty minutes are set aside for you to be examined on short cases. These are usually general medicine or paediatrics. If you saw a paediatric long case you will often get general medicine short cases and vice versa.

The examiners will tell you exactly what they want you to do and you should follow their instructions implicitly. For example, 'examine this praecordium' means look at, palpate and auscultate the chest wall which overlies the heart. Do exactly that. 'Examine the heart' means do a full examination of the cardiovascular system starting at the hands. Some examiners like candidates to 'talk them through' the examination as it is performed. Other examiners do not. You should be prepared to do the examination either way.

The examiners will then ask you questions such as:

— what is the diagnosis?
— what did you think of this murmur?
— what abnormality did you find?

This is often followed up by the questions:

— what are the causes of X?
— what are the associations of X?

It is therefore essential to have a brief list of the causes of any sign or clinical diagnosis. The list should be brief and should include the most common causes first. It is important that these lists are not too long so they are easily at your fingertips. I will say more about this in the later parts of this book.

In psychiatric short cases you must be prepared to do a brief mental state examination on the patient. Alternatively, an increasingly popular way of testing candidates' ability to assess a mental state is by means of video recording. A video is shown of a patient's mental state being assessed. You will then be asked to comment on what you have seen.

The short cases give the examiners a unique chance to see what you are like in a clinical setting. One of the things they are looking for is a professional examination. This can be hard to project under such intense pressure, unless you are on 'automatic pilot'.

The concept of being on 'automatic pilot' is a simple one. You need to practise your examination technique in a pressure setting, preferably with a senior doctor watching. Practise examining any system, organ or anatomical region you can think of. Practise it again and again (under pressure). Eventually you will achieve the dizzy heights of being on 'automatic pilot'. That is, you will not need to think about what bit to examine next (when you are asked to examine a respiratory system for example) because you will do it automatically. You are now free to think about other things during the examination, such as making it look stylish and professional, what are the physical signs, what is the diagnosis, etc.

The examiners will also want to see that you are conventional, competent and have common sense and a caring attitude. Always be polite to the patient. Never hurt the patient. Always make sure he is comfortable. The short cases hold terror for some because you are really on the spot. The patient is in front of you and the examiners want to know the answers. You have little time to think about what you are going to say. It is possible to gain a vital few seconds thinking time in two ways during the short cases.

Firstly, when you are using your stethoscope. You can use this period for extra thinking time. You will have heard the necessary physical signs — you just need a few seconds to think. Leave the stethoscope in position (appearing to be examining) but all the while you have an extra few seconds to gather your thoughts on the case in front of you. This is a particularly useful tip when examining an abdomen, as it is highly unlikely that you will hear abnormal bowel sounds or a bruit in the setting of the short case exam.

Secondly, help the patient to get comfortable after you have finished examining her (for example help her on with her dressing gown). This not only gives an extra second or two's thinking time, but presents a caring attitude to the examiners — they will like it!

I cannot overemphasise the importance of the need to practise. Get a doctor to take a small group of you to see some model short cases prior to the exam. Encourage mutual (constructive) criticism. Practise and practise again. Once you are on 'automatic pilot' there will be no looking back.

The rest of this section of the book (Chapters 3.2–3.12) deals with the types of questions you are likely to be asked, and the types of patients you are likely to meet during your short case exam. I have emphasised the cases which frequently crop up in the final MB clinical examination, and these are denoted by the symbol '★' in the text. I have also briefly mentioned the rarer, more complicated cases which appear occasionally: these are denoted by the symbol '†'. The information contained in these chapters may also, of course, be relevant to the long case section.

3.2

The cardiovascular system (CVS)

THE TYPES OF QUESTIONS ASKED

You will be asked to do one of five things. Do exactly what the examiner asks you to.

(i) Examine the CVS

This implies a full examination of the CVS. The patient should be comfortable on pillows at 45°. Introduce yourself to the patient and ask him if you may examine him. You should start at the hands and work your way up the arms to the face. Then examine the carotid pulse and JVP and then the heart. Do not forget to listen to the bases, feel for a liver edge, and abdominal aortic aneurysm. Feel all the peripheral pulses and for peripheral oedema. Do not forget to listen for bruits (including renal artery) and to feel for radiofemoral delay.

Follow the scheme set out in Table 3.2.1.

(ii) Examine the heart

You should do exactly the same as in (i), starting at the hands. The examiner may stop you and tell you just to listen to the heart, but at least you have demonstrated that you are aware that the examination of the heart starts at the hands.

(iii) Auscultate the heart

Do exactly what you have been told. Forget the hands and peripheral stuff and get your stethoscope plugged in.

Table 3.2.1   Scheme for examination of the CVS

General inspection
Hands
- peripheral cyanosis
- pallor
- clubbing (cyanotic congenital heart disease)
- splinters (infective endocarditis)
- nailfold infarction
- Quincke's sign (capillary pulsation of the nail beds found in aortic incompetence)

Radial pulse (make sure you time it with the second hand of your watch and examine both pulses)
- rate
- rhythm
- character

Radiofemoral delay — coarctation of aorta
Blood pressure
Conjunctivae — anaemia
Mouth — mucosal membranes, central cyanosis or pallor
Carotid pulses (both) — but not at the same time

JVP
Make sure you examine the *internal* jugular vein. The patient's neck must be relaxed. Remember the hepatojugular reflex. If you can't see the top of the JVP, sit the patient up to 90°. Earlobes will waggle if the JVP is very high

Look at the precordium
Scars (previous surgery)
Visible pulsations

Apex beat
Position: you must be seen to assess the exact position in terms of its relationship to the intercostal space (from the angle of Louis) and the mid-clavicular line
Quality
- diffuse (LV dilatation)
- thrusting (LV hypertrophy)
- dyskinetic segment (LV aneurysm)

Palpate precordium
Thrills (palpable murmurs): this is best done over each valvular area with the palm of the hand. The metacarpal heads seem to be the most sensitive area of the hand to use for this
Palpable heart sounds: for all intents and purposes this means feel for the first heart sound of mitral stenosis, which is frequently palpable. It is this which gives the apex beat its 'tapping' quality in this condition (difficult sign)

Auscultation
Murmurs
Third and fourth heart sounds

Table 3.2.1   *(contd)*
Listen over each valvular area in turn with both the bell and diaphragm. Do not forget to turn the patient into the left lateral position and listen to the apex and axilla for mitral murmurs. Always sit the patient forwards and listen in expiration to the aortic area and down the left sternal edge for the murmur of aortic incompetence. Whilst in this position listen for carotid radiation/carotid bruits
Both bases The patient is now sitting up. Take the opportunity to listen to both lung bases for crackles (left ventricular failure)
Abdomen Liver, pulsatile (tricuspid regurgitation) Abdominal aortic aneurysm Renal artery bruits
Legs Peripheral pulses — examine all of them Peripheral oedema

(iv) Examine the pulse

You will usually be offered the right radial. If it is difficult to feel go to the left radial or carotid. Time the pulse with the second hand of your watch. When examining the carotid pulse, do the right carotid artery with the left thumb and the left carotid artery with the right thumb.

The following parameters must be assessed when examining a pulse:

- rate
- rhythm
- character
  - slow rising (aortic stenosis)
  - water hammer (aortic regurgitation)
  - bisferiens (the double-topped pulse found in mixed aortic valve disease).

Occasionally the carotid pulse is visible from the end of the bed in aortic regurgitation (Corrigan's sign). In very severe aortic regurgitation the head may actually nod. This is called De Musset's sign.

(v) Examine the JVP

The patient must be 45° with the head tilted and supported by a pillow to relax the strap muscles of the neck. It is usually best to turn the patient's face towards the left to achieve this. The JVP is best assessed in natural light; this may not be possible in the examination setting. It is essential to assess the internal jugular vein, not the external jugular. The external jugular vein may be raised due to local entrapment in the neck as it passes through the strap muscles and must therefore not be used as an indicator of the central venous pressure.

You need to know how to differentiate the JVP from carotid pulsation. The features to look for are:

- Double impulse in venous pulsation (not present in atrial fibrillation).
- The JVP falls on sitting up (usually). Carotid pulsation will not.
- Hepatojugular reflex. Venous return can be increased by pressing on the liver area. This will cause pulsation in the neck due to the JVP becoming more prominent. This distinguishes it from carotid pulsation.
- Filling from above. The JVP will fill from above when the internal jugular vein is pressed on firmly. Carotid pulsation will not.
- JVP is usually impalpable; the carotid pulsation is usually palpable.
- Level of pulsation in JVP usually falls in inspiration.

A raised JVP may be found in many conditions, but the common ones found in the examination are:

- left ventricular failure
- severe right ventricular failure with tricuspid regurgitation; this may be secondary to valvular heart disease, ischaemic heart disease or cor pulmonale.

TYPICAL CASES

CVS

- Murmurs
- Right-sided murmurs
- Ventricular septal defect
- Atrial septal defect
- Ischaemic heart disease
- Atrial fibrillation
- Left ventricular failure
- Hypertension
- Coarctation of the aorta
- Situs invertus/dextrocardia
- Aortic aneurysm

Cardiovascular short cases are common. This is because valvular heart disease is common (although now becoming less so) and the signs are chronic.

Murmurs* (see Table 3.2.2)

Right-sided murmurs†

- Tricuspid regurgitation
- Pulmonary stenosis
- Pulmonary incompetence
- Tricuspid stenosis

Most people regard these as postgraduate murmurs.

Ventricular septal defect (VSD)†

Rare. Sounds like mitral regurgitation at the left sternal edge (pansystolic, harsh).

Causes

- Congenital (maladie de Roger)

Table 3.2.2 Common final MB murmurs

Murmur	Sign	Associated findings	Causes
Aortic stenosis	Ejection systolic murmur which radiates to carotids	Slow rising pulse Heaving apex Low systolic BP LVH on ECG and CXR	Congenital (bifid valve) Rheumatic
Aortic incompetence (regurgitation)	Blowing early diastolic murmur (aortic area or LSE with patient sitting up in expiration)	Water-hammer pulse Wide pulse pressure Corrigan's sign De Musset's sign Quincke's sign Heaving apex LVH on ECG and CXR	Rheumatic Dissecting aortic aneurysm Ankylosing spondylitis Marfan's syndrome Congenital Syphilis
Mitral stenosis	Rumbling mid-diastolic murmur at apex	Palpable first heart sound Presystolic accentuation if patient in sinus rhythm AF Opening snap	Usually rheumatic
Mitral incompetence	Pansystolic murmur at apex	Radiates to axilla, best heard left lateral position	Rheumatic LV dilatation (any cause) Ruptured chordae, etc.

NB: *Aortic sclerosis* has exactly the same murmur as *aortic stenosis*, but none of the associated physical findings. It is due to thickening of the aortic valve (calcific age-related change) and is of no import, save that it has to be distinguished from aortic stenosis.

- Post-MI (septal rupture — this is very rare in an exam as the patients are too sick).

Atrial septal defect (ASD)†

Rare. Fixed splitting of first heart sound with a pulmonary systolic flow murmur (postgraduate murmur).

Cause

- Congenital.

Ischaemic heart disease

Common long case (angina or post-myocardial infarction). Uncommon short case. History very important:

- cardiac pain
- past medical history of hypertension, diabetes or hyperlipidaemia
- family history
- smoking.

Signs

The patient may have no signs but look for xanthelasmata, hypertension, signs of diabetes, signs of left ventricular dysfunction. The ECG may be normal.

Atrial fibrillation*

Very common.

Signs

Irregularly irregular pulse. No 'a' waves in JVP (distinguishes it from multiple VEs, which can also cause an irregularly irregular pulse). ECG shows irregular QRS complex with no 'P' waves (see p. 179)

Causes

- Ischaemic heart disease*
- Post-myocardial infarction*

- Mitral stenosis*
- Thyrotoxicosis
- Pulmonary embolism
- ASD
- Hypertensive heart disease
- Malignant infiltration of pericardium.

Left ventricular failure

Although this is a very common diagnosis in everyday clinical practice, it is not often included in the examination. The reason for this is that patients with acute left ventricular failure are too unwell to be included. You may get someone in the recovery phase, but by this stage the signs will be disappearing or have gone altogether.

Signs

- Tachypnoea
- Central cyanosis
- Sinus tachycardia
- Raised JVP
- Third heart sound
- Crackles at both bases.

ECG shows left ventricular strain pattern. CXR shows cardiomegaly, upper lobe blood diversion, interstitial shadowing, Kerley B lines, bat's wing appearance (see p. 205)

Hypertension

Common long case. Less common short case.

Ninety percent of the cases are primary*. Ten percent are secondary to:

- renal disease*
- coarctation
- Cushing's disease
- Conn's syndrome
- acromegaly
- phaeochromocytoma.

Signs

Look for the effects of hypertension on the:

- Eyes
  — a-v nipping
  — increased vessel tortuosity
  — haemorrhage
  — exudates
  — papilloedema
- Heart — signs of LVH, ischaemic heart disease
- Kidneys — signs of chronic renal failure
- Peripheral vasculature.

You need to know a little bit about the investigations and the treatment of hypertension. These are commonly asked questions.

Coarctation of the aorta[†]

This is a very rare cause of hypertension.

Signs

- Radio-femoral delay.
- You can sometimes hear odd murmurs on the upper chest and back due to blood flow through the collaterals.
- Hypertension in the arms, hypotension in the legs.
- CXR (see p. 208)
  — rib notching
  — post-stenotic dilatation of aorta.

Situs invertus/dextrocardia[†]

This is very very rare, but much loved by the examiners.

Causes

Dextrocardia is one of the few causes of inaudible heart sounds. Other causes are:

- obesity[*]
- chronic obstructive airways disease[*]
- left pleural effusion (large)
- pericardial effusion
- stethoscope not adjusted properly[*].

If you think your patient has dextrocardia, other organs could also be transposed. There is an association with Kartaganer's syndrome.

Aortic aneurysm

- Abdominal — this is really a surgical case.
- Thoracic[†] — the patient will complain of back and chest pain or a hoarse voice; signs include a tracheal tug and aortic regurgitation.

Causes

- Syphilis
- Atheroma
- Post-dissection of aorta
- Traumatic.

KEY QUESTIONS

CVS

1. **What are the causes of:**
   - atrial fibrillation
   - sinus tachycardia
   - sinus bradycardia
   - a raised JVP
   - aortic regurgitation
   - aortic stenosis
   - mitral regurgitation
   - mitral stenosis
   - left ventricular failure
   - an impalpable apex
   - hypertension?
2. **What are the risk factors associated with ischaemic heart disease?**
3. **How can you tell the difference clinically between:**
   - a raised JVP and a visible carotid pulsation
   - the murmur of aortic regurgitation and mitral stenosis
   - the murmur of mitral regurgitation and aortic stenosis
   - aortic stenosis and aortic sclerosis?

3.3

The respiratory system

The standard question in the short cases is: 'Examine this patient's chest/respiratory system'. This should be done quickly but professionally. The patient should be comfortable, propped up by pillows at 45°. Introduce yourself. Ask permission to examine the patient. The guide for examination of the respiratory system is set out in Table 3.3.1.

Table 3.3.1

General inspection
Respiratory rate
Hands
- clubbing (bronchial carcinoma)
- nicotine staining (COAD, bronchial carcinoma)
- CO_2 retention flap (respiratory failure)
- essential tremor (β_2 agonist therapy)
- peripheral cyanosis
Pulse
Conjunctivae — suffusion (polycythaemia in COAD, or SVC obstruction)
Anaemia
Mucosae of mouth — central cyanosis
Trachea position — think of things which push (pleural effusion) or pull (collapse) to one side
Nodes
- supraclavicular
- cervical
- occipital
- axillary
   Supraclavicular nodes are best felt from behind to allow the fingertips to get right in behind the clavicles

JVP
Raised in cor pulmonale and SVC obstruction

Table 3.3.1   (*contd*)

Apex beat
Determine the position exactly. This will, together with the tracheal position, allow you to determine if there is any mediastinal shift. If the apex beat is impalpable, this is also useful information, e.g. COAD

Right ventricular heave
Cor pulmonale

Expansion
This is arguably the most important sign in chest medicine. It is done quite badly and is quite tricky to do well. Get an experienced doctor to show you how. It tells you where the pathology is (pathology = side with least expansion). It is bilaterally decreased in COAD

— *Percussion*
— *Auscultation*   Compare right with
— *Tactile vocal fremitus*   left on front of
— *Auditory resonance*   chest.

   Now you need to sit the patient forward and repeat the above examination from 'expansion' on the back of the chest

Whispering pectoriloquy
This is an over-rated clinical sign. The way to elicit it is to get the patient to whisper 'one, one, one'. The sounds are heard better over an area of consolidation or the top of a pleural effusion

Examine the ankles for pitting oedema (cor pulmonale?)

Sputum pot
Do not forget to look for it. It may give an important clue to the diagnosis, e.g. haemoptysis

CXR
Ask to see it

TYPICAL CASES

THE RESPIRATORY SYSTEM

- Clubbing
- Carcinoma of lung
- Chronic obstructive airways disease
- Asthma
- Pleural effusion

continued

- Fibrosing alveolitis
- Pneumothorax
- Sarcoidosis
- Haemoptysis
- Thoracoplasty/physical treatments for TB
- Superior vena cava obstruction
- Cor pulmonale
- Pneumonia
- Bronchiectasis

Clubbing*

Very common short case.

Causes

- Familial
- Idiopathic
- Carcinoma of the bronchus*
- Chronic suppurative lung disease
  — cystic fibrosis
  — empyema
  — bronchiectasis
  — lung abscess
- Fibrosing alveolitis
- Congenital cyanotic heart disease
- Infective endocarditis
- Cirrhosis of liver†
- Ulcerative colitis†
- Crohn's disease†.

You *must* know this list.

Carcinoma of lung*

Very common case.

Signs

Look for:

- cachexia
- clubbing

- nicotine-stained fingers
- lymph nodes
- signs of intrathoracic involvement, for example:
  — pleural effusion
  — collapse
  — recurrent chest infections.

Ask to see the chest X-ray and sputum pot.

Remember Pancoast's tumour. This is a carcinoma of the bronchus at the apex causing an ipsilateral Horner's syndrome (involvement of sympathetic chain) and ipsilateral wasting of the small muscles of the hand (T1 root of brachial plexus involved).

Chronic obstructive airways disease*

Common case.

Signs

- Nicotine-stained fingers
- CO_2 retention flap (rare in the exam)
- β_2 agonist tremor
- Tachypnoea
- Pursed lip breathing   } 'pink puffer'
- Using accessory muscles of respiration
- Centrally cyanosed   } 'blue bloater'
- Peripheral oedema
- Overexpansion/barrel-shaped chest
- Hyperresonant percussion note
- Loss of cardiac dullness
- Impalpable apex beat
- Distant heart sounds
- Wheeze/reduced air entry.

You need to know about the aetiology, treatment and chest X-ray appearance. Patients have an obstructive deficit on respiratory function testing with an FEV_1/FVC ratio of less than 0.75.

Asthma

Acute asthma will not appear in the examination for obvious reasons. A patient in the recovery phase from an acute attack or a patient with the more chronic variety is sometimes included.

Signs

There may be none. The patient may be overexpanded or there may be wheeze in the chest. Ask to look at the peak flow chart.

From Figure 3.3.1 you ought to note that the patient has morning dips and that there is a gradual increase in the peak flow as the patient recovers. In addition to this there is also a gradual reduction in the diurnal variation in peak flow as the patient recovers. Figure 3.3.2 shows a peak flow recorded in chronic asthma. Again note the morning dips around the average of 300 l/min.

You need to know about the assessment and treatment of acute severe asthma (see p. 230).

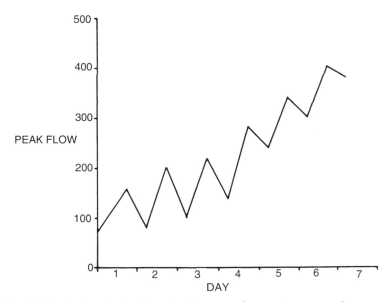

Fig. 3.3.1   Peak expiratory flow rate of recovery from acute severe asthma. Note that the morning 'dipping' improves as the patient recovers.

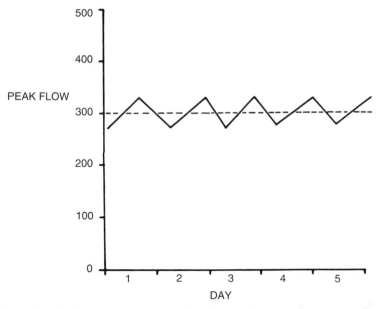

Fig. 3.3.2 Peak expiratory flow chart of stable chronic asthma.

Pleural effusion

This will usually crop up if there happens to be a patient with a pleural effusion on the ward at the time of the exam. Chronic pleural effusion in out-patients is uncommon.

Signs

- Reduced expansion.
- Stony, dull percussion note.
- Absent breath sounds.
- There may be bronchial breathing and/or whispering pectoriloquy over the top of the effusion.
- Mediastinum may be shifted away from the side of the effusion, if it is a large one.
- Signs of previous pleural tap, e.g. sticking plaster on patient's back.

Causes

1. Exudate — protein content greater than 30 g/l.
2. Transudate — protein content less than 30 g/l.

Exudate

- Neoplastic
  - secondary pleural deposits, e.g. from lung or breast*
  - primary mesothelioma
- Inflammatory — following pneumonia*
  - bacterial
  - viral
  - tubercle
- Pulmonary embolus
- Trauma
- Rheumatoid arthritis, SLE
- Subphrenic abscess, pancreatitis.

Transudate

- Heart failure*
- Cirrhosis of liver*

- Nephrotic syndrome
- Meig's syndrome.

Fibrosing alveolitis

Although this condition is not that common, the signs are chronic and such patients are frequently included.

Signs

- Clubbing
- Central cyanosis
- Reduced expansion (bilateral)
- Bilateral fine inspiratory crackles worse at bases.

Causes

- Idiopathic*
- Rheumatoid arthritis
- SLE
- Asbestosis.

The idiopathic variety often responds to steroids, so look for the Cushingoid appearance and easy bruising.

Chest X-ray shows reduced lung volumes and fluffy shadows, which start at the bases and work upwards. They make the heart border and diaphragm indistinct.

Respiratory function shows a restrictive deficit with FEV_1/FVC greater than 75% and the vital capacity will invariably be reduced.

Pneumothorax†

This is a very rare exam case.

Sarcoidosis†

Rare short case. Sometimes included in the long cases.

Signs

- Erythema nodosum
- Bilateral hilar lymphadenopathy on chest X-ray
- Bilateral uveitis
- Chest examination is often normal.

It can also cause (rarely) hepatomegaly, splenomegaly, skin deposits, VII nerve palsies (sometimes bilateral), diffuse CNS involvement. There is often a restrictive defect on the respiratory function tests with an FEV_1/FVC greater than 75% and a reduced transfer factor. If the patient is asymptomatic no treatment is indicated. If the patient is symptomatic, or has widespread disease or worsening transfer factor/X-ray, they should be treated with prednisolone.

Haemoptysis

You will occasionally be asked: 'Examine this patient who has been coughing up blood'. More commonly you will find blood in the sputum pot (if you remember to look in it) during the course of your examination.

Causes

Think of the following causes:

- pneumonia (bacterial)*
- tuberculosis*
- carcinoma of the lung*
- bronchiectasis
- mitral stenosis
- post-traumatic
- pulmonary embolus
- idiopathic (this is a common cause in young people in everyday practice, but not in the exam).

Thoracoplasty/physical treatments for TB[†]

Patients treated for tuberculosis up until the early 1950s used to have quite drastic surgical procedures as part of their management. They are becoming increasingly scarce as this cohort of patients ages. They are sometimes brought up for the exam.

Signs

- Thoracoplasty
- Ping pong balls — inserted into upper pleural space to maintain an artificial pneumothorax.

Superior vena cava obstruction[†]

This is rare as an examination case, but you need to look for plethora of the upper half of the body and conjunctival suffusion, fixed raised JVP, swelling of the arms, face and neck, and collateral vessels. The usual cause is carcinoma of the bronchus impinging on the superior vena cava. It is a 'radiotherapy emergency'. Look for marks on the chest to see if the patient has had or is having a course of radiotherapy.

Cor pulmonale

Students often get confused about this. Any chest condition causing prolonged hypoxia will eventually cause pulmonary hypertension. This is due to a direct effect of hypoxia on the pulmonary microcirculation. The pulmonary hypertension, in turn, causes a strain on the right side of the heart. This results in right ventricular hypertrophy and, eventually, right ventricular failure.

Signs

- Central cyanosis
- Right ventricular heave (felt with the flat of the hand at the left sternal edge)
- Raised JVP
- Peripheral oedema (pitting)
- There may also be hepatomegaly.

You need to remember to look for the causes of the cor pulmonale, e.g. chronic obstructive airways disease or fibrosing alveolitis.

Pneumonia

Cases of pneumonia in the final MB are uncommon. However, you may get a patient in the recovery phase.

Signs

You will need to look for signs of consolidation/collapse when examining the chest. The patient may have residual fever.

Causes

There are many causes of pneumonia but remember the following headings:

1. Bacterial, e.g. *Streptococcus pneumoniae, Haemophilus influenzae,* tuberculosis, *Klebsiella, Staphylococcus.*
2. Viral, including *cytomegalovirus, influenza virus, RSV, adenovirus,* etc.
3. Rare causes, such as *Pneumocystis carinii,* yeasts and fungi (immunocompromised patient).

Mycoplasma can cause pneumonia in otherwise fit adults.

Bronchiectasis

Signs

- Clubbing of fingernails
- Late inspiratory crackles (often unilateral).

Sputum pot will show purulent, thick secretions and may also contain blood. The pathogenesis involves local dilatation of the bronchi with subsequent collection of purulent secretions.

Causes

- Tuberculosis
- Measles
- Post-nasal drip
- Foreign body
- Post-pneumonia
- Cystic fibrosis
- Idiopathic.

There is an association with Kartaganer's syndrome. This is a combination of post-nasal drip, bronchiectasis and infertility. This is due to an abnormality of cilial function. Occasionally, situs invertus or dextrocardia is found in this syndrome.

KEY QUESTIONS

THE RESPIRATORY SYSTEM

1. **What are the causes of:**
   - clubbing of the finger nails
   - pleural effusion
   - haemoptysis
   - primary community-acquired chest infections
   - bronchiectasis
   - cor pulmonale?
2. **How would you differentiate clinically between**
   - consolidation and collapse
   - pneumothorax and pleural effusion
   - peripheral and central cyanosis
   - restrictive and obstructive airways disease?
3. **Define central cyanosis.**
4. **What respiratory problems are encountered in patients with HIV-related disease?**

Table 3.3.2 Signs in respiratory disease. You may find the following table helpful to sort out what is going on inside the chest when you are examining it

	Mediastinum	Expansion	Percussion note	Breath sounds	Tactile vocal fremitus
Pleural effusion	Moves away from affected side	→	Stony dull	Absent	→
Pneumothorax	No difference (away from affected side if tension)	→	Hyperresonant	Absent	→
Collapse	Towards affected side	→	→	↓ or ↑ if associated consolidation	→
Consolidation	No change Towards affected side if associated collapse	→	→	↑ or bronchial breathing/whispering pectoriloquy	←

Note (i) Collapse and consolidation often coexist in real life, and so the signs are mixed.
 (ii) Bronchial breathing and whispering pectoriloquy can be heard above a pleural effusion (sometimes).

3.4

The gastrointestinal tract (GIT)

The GIT should be examined in a thorough, systematic way. It is important not to hurt the patient, and before you start your examination you should always ask if the patient has any tenderness in the abdomen. During the course of the examination it is essential to keep glancing at the patient's face, to ensure that you are not causing any discomfort. The other advantage of asking the patient if she has any pain or tenderness in the abdomen is that, if she has, the location of this tenderness may give an important clue as to the site of the pathology. For example, if the patient says she is tender in the right upper quadrant, the chances are that she has tender hepatomegaly.

The usual question asked in the short case is either to examine the GIT or examine the abdomen. This essentially means a full examination of the GIT, starting at the hands, as set out in Table 3.4.1. Occasionally you will be asked just to 'palpate the abdomen'. In this case, do exactly what you are told, and no more. However, do not forget to use your eyes, e.g. if you see a fullness in the left hypochondrium, make sure you feel particularly thoroughly for a spleen.

The patient should be laid flat in bed. If she is uncomfortable without a pillow, one should be provided. Traditionally the area from knees to nipples should be exposed, but in the exam setting the patient's modesty should be preserved, so the lower limit of exposure should be just above the pubis.

The general scheme for the examination of the GIT is set out in Table 3.4.1.

SPECIFIC POINTS TO NOTE ON GIT EXAMINATION

Observation of abdomen

Ask the patient to take a deep breath in whilst observing the abdomen. This accentuates areas of fullness caused by underlying

Table 3.4.1   Scheme for examination of the GIT

General inspection
Wasting, scars, etc.

Hands
Clubbing (cirrhosis, Crohn's disease)
Palmar erythema, Dupuytren's contracture, leuconychia (chronic liver disease)

Liver flap
Hepatic encephalopathy

Conjunctivae
Jaundice, anaemia

Mouth
Telangiectasia (hereditary haemorrhagic telangiectasia)
Perioral pigmentation (Peutz–Jegher syndrome)

Tongue

Supraclavicular nodes
Virchow's node, Troisier's sign

Skin on chest wall
Spider naevi, gynaecomastia, bruising/purpura (chronic liver disease)

Observation of abdomen
Areas of fullness
• masses
• organomegaly
• ascites
Scars (see Fig. 3.4.1)
Distended veins on the anterior abdominal wall. Determine direction of blood flow (see Fig. 3.4.2)
Everted umbilicus (ascites; several litres of fluid needed to produce this sign)

Palpation
Light and deep, do each quadrant in turn
Feel for masses, organomegaly (liver, kidneys, spleen, bladder, uterus) and tenderness. Remember to look at the patient's face

Percussion
Areas of dullness corresponding to masses/organomegaly

Shifting dullness/fluid thrill

Auscultation
Bowel sounds — bruits (renal artery, aortic, hepatic)
'Liver scratch sign' (Fig. 3.4.3)
Extra thinking time (see Chapter 1.1)

Hernial orifices

Peripheral oedema

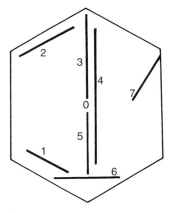

Fig. 3.4.1   Abdominal scars.
1 Appendix. 2 Cholecystectomy. 3 Gastric surgery. 4 Laparotomy.
5 Hysterectomy/Classical Caesarian. 6 Caesarian section. 7 Nephrectomy.

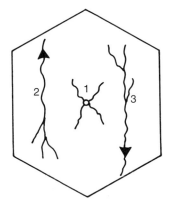

Fig. 3.4.2   Abnormal anterior abdominal veins. 1 *Caput medusae*; dilated
veins around the umbilicus, found in portal hypertension: flow is away from the
umbilicus. 2 *IVC obstruction*: flow upwards. 3 *SVC obstruction*: flow downwards.

organomegaly/masses. Now ask the patient to raise her feet off the
bed whilst you observe the abdomen. Any lurking incisional herniae
or divarification of the recti will now be obvious.

Palpation

Palpation should be performed from the patient's left side whilst
kneeling or sitting. The reason for this is that the hand is more

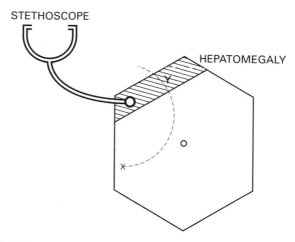

Fig. 3.4.3 The liver scratch sign. This technique is helpful to confirm the presence of hepatomegaly, suspected by palpation and percussion. It is particularly useful in the obese patient, when percussion and palpation of organs may be difficult. Listen with the stethoscope over the liver edge. At the same time lightly scratch the abdominal wall with the fingernail in the right iliac fossa (point X). Work your way upwards, scratching gently as you go but keeping your finger at the same distance from the stethoscope at all times. When you come over the liver edge (point Y), you will hear a loud scratching noise. This is because the scratching sound is being transmitted through the liver substance, which is solid and therefore a good sound conductor.

relaxed and more in contact with the patient in this position. It is far more sensitive than examining the patient whilst you are in the standing position.

Liver

Start in the right iliac fossa (RIF) and work upwards, asking the patient to breathe in as you palpate.

Spleen

Start in the RIF and work towards the left hypochondrium. If you start in the left iliac fossa (LIF) or left hypochondrium you may miss a very large spleen. To feel a small spleen it may be necessary to get the patient to roll partly onto the right side and feel with the fingertips under the left costal margin (during inspiration). The spleen needs to be enlarged to at least twice its normal size for it to be palpable.

Percussion

Percuss the whole abdomen. Remember to percuss the upper border of the liver and spleen.

Ascites

Shifting dullness

Percuss out the anterior limit of the fluid level. This is best done with your finger parallel to the air/fluid interface (i.e. in the sagittal plane). Now ask the patient to roll onto their side. Re-percuss to assess if the area of dullness has moved, which indicates free fluid in the peritoneal space.

Fluid thrill

If you have demonstrated shifting dullness, go on to try to demonstrate a fluid thrill. Ask the examiner to firmly place the hypothenar aspect of his hand on the midline of the anterior abdominal wall (in the sagittal plane). Flick the fluid at one side, whilst palpating the other.

PR/genitals

Do not examine the genitals or perform a rectal examination, but express the desirability of doing so.

TYPICAL CASES

GIT

- Hepatomegaly
- Splenomegaly
- Hepatosplenomegaly
- Ascites
- Mass in the abdomen
- Jaundice
- Anaemia
- Chronic liver disease
- Carcinoid syndrome
- Other cases

Hepatomegaly*

Delineate the lower border of the liver, and size it in terms of finger breadths below the costal margin. Remember also to find where the upper border is (by percussion). This is important because occasionally a liver edge can be felt just below the costal margin when there is no true hepatomegaly, e.g. chronic obstructive airways disease where hyperexpanded lungs push down the (normal-sized) liver.

Define the characteristics of the liver edge you have felt in terms of:

- the edge
  - smooth
  - knobbly (multiple metastases)
- pulsatility (tricuspid regurgitation)
- consistency
  - firm
  - hard
- bruit (hepatocellular carcinoma, a-v malformation)
- tenderness (hepatitis, capsular pain of the hepatomegaly of congestive cardiac failure).

Think of the causes of hepatomegaly and look for other signs which may give you the diagnosis of the patient in front of you (see Table 3.4.2).

Table 3.4.2 Hepatomegaly: causes and signs to look for	
Cause	Signs to look for
Chronic liver disease* (of any aetiology)	See p. 71
Fatty infiltration* Congestive cardiac failure (CCF)	Alcohol abuse (may be no other signs) ↑ JVP Signs of LVF • crackles at the bases • third heart sound
Metastatic carcinoma	Look for the site of primary • breasts • lung • prostate, etc.
Hepatitis† (A, B, C)	Jaundice, splenomegaly, tattoos, signs of i.v. drug abuse Ask about travel, transfusions, sexual history
Hepatoma†	Listen for bruit Ask about past history of hepatitis B or C, cirrhosis

Table 3.4.2 (*Contd*)

Cause	Signs to look for
Lymphoma[†]	Splenomegaly, lymphadenopathy, fever, weight loss
Leukaemia (all types)[†]	Splenomegaly, nodes (CLL), purpura, petechiae, fever, etc.

Notes:
(1) In the later stages of cirrhosis the liver may be impalpable, as it is small, shrunken and fibrosed.
(2) Very rare exam cases: sarcoid; TB, infectious mononucleosis (EB virus, CMV, toxoplasmosis), RA, SLE.

Splenomegaly*

A favourite examiners' question is 'how can you tell the difference clinically between splenomegaly and a palpable left kidney?'

Answer

The spleen has a notch, whereas a kidney does not. You can ballot a kidney but you cannot ballot a spleen. A spleen is dull to percussion, a kidney is not. You cannot get above a spleen, but you sometimes can get above a kidney. (I never have, except a transplanted or horse-shoe kidney.)

Categories of splenomegaly

Splenomegaly is subjectively categorised as mild, moderate or large:

- Large (past umbilicus)
  - chronic granulocytic leukaemia
  - myelofibrosis
  - kala-azar[†] (*not* in UK).
- Moderate (up to the umbilicus)
  - lymphoma
  - chronic lymphatic leukaemia (CLL)
  - portal hypertension
  - malaria[†].
- Mild (just palpable)
  - portal hypertension (of any cause)
  - lymphoma
  - CLL
  - polycythaemia rubra vera

—rheumatoid arthritis (ask to see full blood count result —
Felty's syndrome)
— SLE ⎫
— amyloidosis ⎪
— hepatitis ⎬ Rare in the exam
— infectious mononucleosis ⎪
— malaria. ⎭

Hepatosplenomegaly*

Causes

- Chronic liver disease (of any cause) with portal hypertension*
- Lymphoma
- Leukaemia (any type)
- Infections[†]
  — hepatitis (A, B, C)
  — infectious mononucleosis, TB
- Amyloid[†]
- Sarcoid[†]
- SLE.

Ascites

You need to examine for this in the correct manner, as described
earlier in the chapter. Fullness in both flanks on general inspection
usually gives the game away (the only other common cause for
this is polycystic disease of the kidneys). Look for an everted
umbilicus.

Causes

The commonest cause, by far, is cirrhosis of the liver. It is helpful
to think of the causes of ascites under the following headings:

- hypoalbuminaemia
  — chronic liver disease (any cause)*
  — protein–calorie malnutrition
  — nephrotic syndrome
  — protein-losing enteropathy
- portal hypertension — chronic liver disease*
- local inflammatory process

— metastatic carcinoma (in the peritoneum)
— pelvic carcinoma (ovary)
— infection (e.g. peritoneal TB).

Mass in the abdomen

This is not a particularly common case, as it is really 'surgical'. The patient can often help you, if you let her. Remember to ask if she is tender anywhere. If she is, ask her where her tenderness is. This may well be of considerable help in localising the pathology.

Causes

The causes of a mass in the abdomen depend on the location of the mass:

- RUQ
  - gallbladder
  - carcinoma head of pancreas
  - Reidel's lobe
  - right kidney
  - carcinoma colon (hepatic flexure)
- epigastrium
  - carcinoma stomach
  - enlarged left lobe liver
  - pancreatic pseudocyst
  - pancreatic carcinoma
  - abdominal aortic aneurysm
- LUQ
  - spleen
  - left kidney
  - carcinoma splenic flexure
  - carcinoma tail of pancreas
- central/periumbilical
  - abdominal aortic aneurysm
  - carcinoma body of pancreas
  - pancreatic pseudocyst
- RIF
  - carcinoma caecum
  - right ovarian mass
  - mass of matted small bowel (e.g. Crohn's)

- LIF
  — carcinoma sigmoid colon
  — left ovarian mass
  — transplanted kidney.

Jaundice

The patient will almost invariably be an in-patient. This fact makes jaundice an uncommon examination case.

Causes

Remember the basic causes:

- Pre-hepatic
  — autoimmune haemolytic anaemia
  — drug-induced haemolytic anaemia (e.g. methyldopa)
  — hereditary spherocytosis
  — sickle cell anaemia
  — thalassaemias
  — transfusion reactions
  — red cell fragmentation syndromes (e.g. DIC secondary to septicaemia)
  — Gilbert's syndrome*.
- Hepatic
  — chronic liver disease (any cause)
  — acute hepatitis (A, B, C, glandular fever, Weil's disease)†
  — metastatic carcinoma of the liver
  — hepatotoxic drugs (e.g. post-paracetamol overdose, halothane).
- Cholestasis
  — drugs, e.g. chlorpromazine
  — biliary obstruction
  — gallstones
  — carcinoma of pancreas
  — primary sclerosing cholangitis (PSC).

It can be difficult or impossible to distinguish between these causes clinically. Points to look out for which may give a clue are found in the patient's history, the examination, and the investigation (see below).

History

- Transfusions
- Travel
- Tattoos   } Hepatitis B and C
- Drug abuse (intravenous)
- Sexual preferences
- Infectious contacts
- Job (sewers) — Weil's disease[†]
- Family history of jaundice or splenectomy (suggests haemolysis)
- Past history of recurrent jaundice
  — haemolysis
  — Gilbert's syndrome
- Drug history (see above)
- Alcohol intake
- Back/abdominal pains (pancreatitis/carcinoma of pancreas)
- Ulcerative colitis/fever/jaundice — PSC.

Examination

Look for:

- stigmata of chronic liver disease
- hepatomegaly (knobbly in secondary carcinoma)
- splenomegaly (haemolysis or portal hypertension)
- anaemia (haemolysis)
- palpable gallbladder (carcinoma of pancreas)
- needle puncture marks (hepatitis B and C).

Patients with haemolytic jaundice have a lemon yellow tinge.

Investigations

- Raised unconjugated bilirubin
- Urobilinogen in urine   } Imply haemolytic jaundice
- Reduced haptoglobins.

Remember the Coombe's test, Hb electrophoresis and red cell fragility studies.

The ALT and AST are raised out of proportion to the alkaline phosphatase in hepatic jaundice.

Alkaline phosphatase is raised out of proportion to ALT in cholestasis. Ultrasound examination is essential to determine the calibre of the common bile duct. If this is dilated it implies a surgical (cholestatic) cause for the jaundice.

Anaemia

This is unlikely to be the sole sign in a short case and you will usually meet an anaemic patient as a long case. The causes are listed in Table 3.4.3.

Table 3.4.3 Causes of anaemia

Hypochromic microcytic
Iron deficiency due to:
Chronic blood loss
* peptic ulcer
* carcinoma of the stomach, colon or caecum
* colitis
* uterine
* renal tract
Malabsorption secondary to partial gastrectomy, extensive ileal resection, coeliac disease
Dietary
During pregnancy

Normochromic normocytic
Chronic disease
* rheumatoid arthritis
* systemic lupus erythematosus
* Crohn's disease
* carcinoma
* lymphoma
* chronic infections, e.g. TB

Macrocytic
B12 deficiency
* pernicious anaemia
* gastrectomy
* blind-loop syndrome
* tropical sprue
* ileal resection
* Crohn's disease
* dietary (veganism)
Folate deficiency
* dietary (alcoholics, old age, pregnancy)
* malabsorption (see above)
* increased utilisation of folate (pregnancy, haemolysis, myelosclerosis, carcinoma)
* anticonvulsant therapy

Chronic liver disease*

This is a common short case, as chronic liver disease is common and it produces interesting, stable clinical signs. The clinical signs, complications and causes of chronic liver disease are shown in Table 3.4.4.

When you see a patient with signs suggestive of chronic liver disease always check for signs of complications such as portal

---

Table 3.4.4 Signs, complications and causes of chronic liver disease

Signs
Palmar erythema, Dupuytren's
Spider naevi
Gynaecomastia
Testicular atrophy
Hepatomegaly
Ascites
Peripheral oedema
Jaundice
Muscle wasting
Clubbing of the fingernails[†]

Complications
Portal hypertension
• splenomegaly
• ascites
• abnormal abdominal veins
• oesophageal varices
Hepatic encephalopathy
• liver flap
• hepatic foetor
• mental obtundation
Gram-negative sepsis
Primary hepatocellular carcinoma (bruit over liver)

Causes
Common
• alcohol
• chronic hepatitis B, C
• autoimmune chronic active hepatitis
• primary biliary cirrhosis (PBC)
• cryptogenic
Uncommon
• primary sclerosing cholangitis (PSC)
• haemachromatosis
• α_1 antitrypsin deficiency
• Wilson's disease

hypertension, hepatic encephalopathy or a primary liver cancer. It is usually not possible to make an accurate diagnosis as to the aetiology of the chronic liver disease from the clinical examination alone (a liver biopsy is usually required for this). However, there may be clues which suggest the diagnosis:

- i.v. puncture marks, young female
  — hepatitis B, C; autoimmune chronic active hepatitis
- middle-aged female with xanthelasmata
  — primary biliary cirrhosis (PBC)
- ileostomy in a middle-aged male
  — primary sclerosing cholangitis (associated with ulcerative colitis)
- pigmentation
  — haemachromatosis
- Kaiser Fleischer rings
  — Wilson's disease.

Carcinoid syndrome

Very rare in clinical practice. Not quite so rare in the exam.

Signs

- Hepatomegaly (knobbly, due to secondary deposits)
- Facial flushing
- Borborygmi.

The classical patient with carcinoid syndrome gives a history of flushing, diarrhoea and borborygmi. It is caused by release of 5HIAA into the systemic circulation from the secondary deposits in the liver. The primary is usually in the small bowel, appendix, duodenum or pancreas. The reason that patients with carcinoid syndrome do come up as short cases with a certain amount of regularity is that the natural history of the disease (even with secondary deposits in the liver) is often between 10 and 15 years.

Other cases

Other more common chronic gastrointestinal diseases such as peptic ulceration, coeliac disease, Crohn's disease and ulcerative colitis do not come up very often in the short cases, as they often do not have any signs. You may meet them in the long cases.

KEY QUESTIONS

GIT

1. **What are the causes of:**
   - ascites
   - hepatomegaly
   - splenomegaly
   - hepatosplenomegaly
   - liver bruit
   - cirrhosis
   - jaundice
   - diarrhoea
   - constipation
   - anaemia
     — hypochromic microcytic
     — normochromic normocytic
     — megaloblastic
   - macrocytosis (without anaemia)?
2. **What are the signs of chronic liver disease?**
3. **What is the difference clinically between splenomegaly and an enlarged left kidney?**
4. **What clinical signs might you find in a patient with chronic, active inflammatory bowel disease?**

3.5

Renal medicine

Renal medicine is regarded by some as a postgraduate subject. Having said this, on occasion you will meet a renal patient in finals. However, there are only a very limited selection of cases that you are likely to encounter. The likelihood of coming across renal cases in finals varies up and down the country. It essentially depends on your teaching hospital's access to renal patients, dialysis centres, etc. Ask colleagues about what has happened in previous years, as the pattern is likely to repeat itself.

You need to know how to examine the kidneys, and how to distinguish between an enlarged left kidney and an enlarged spleen (see p. 65).

TYPICAL CASES

RENAL MEDICINE

- Polycystic kidneys
- Bilateral renal enlargement
- Unilateral enlarged kidney
- Chronic renal failure

Polycystic kidneys*

This is the commonest renal case in finals.

Clinical features

- Bilaterally palpable kidneys, which feel lobulated (multiple cysts)

- Hypertension
- Signs of chronic renal failure (see later)
- Examine urine for blood/protein/casts
- Ask about the family history.

Polycystic disease of the kidneys is an autosomal dominant condition. There are multiple cysts in the kidneys (and sometimes liver). Patients develop chronic renal failure during adult life and are usually on some form of renal support (dialysis/transplant) by their 40s.

Complications

- Hypertension
- Recurrent urinary tract infections
- Haemorrhage into a cyst
- Ruptured Berry aneurysm (Berry aneurysms are more common in polycystic disease).

Bilateral renal enlargement

Causes

- Polycystic kidneys*
- Bilateral hydronephrosis
- Amyloidosis[†].

Unilateral enlarged kidney

Causes

- Hydronephrosis
- Renal carcinoma
- Simple renal cysts (benign)
- Hypertrophy of single kidney
- Transplanted kidney (left iliac fossa, usually).

Chronic renal failure

You are more likely to meet this as a long case. It is sometimes seen as a short case.

Symptoms

- Malaise
- Tiredness
- Bone pain (osteomalacia), etc.

Signs

- Brown line on fingernails
- Yellow coloration to skin
- Anaemia (reduced erythropoietin production)
- Hypertension
- Signs of fluid overload (raised JVP, peripheral oedema)
- Signs of renal support
  - fistula ⎫
  - shunt ⎬ haemodialysis
  - peritoneal dialysis
  - renal transplant.

You need to look for signs which may tell you the cause of the patient's chronic renal failure.

Causes

- Glomerulonephritis
- Pyelonephritis
- Diabetes
- Hypertension
- Polycystic disease of the kidneys.

3.6

Endocrinology

Endocrinology cases are straightforward, so long as you have prepared yourself properly for them. You will appreciate that there is no particular organ system to examine: your examination should be tailored to the patient in front of you, and may involve examining parts of several 'systems'.

TYPICAL CASES

ENDOCRINOLOGY

- The diabetic
- Hyperthyroidism
- Goitre
- Hypothyroidism
- Acromegaly
- Cushing's syndrome
- Addison's disease
- Hypopituitarism
- Phaeochromocytoma

The diabetic*

It would be unusual for you not to come across a diabetic patient at some stage in the exam. Diabetics are either insulin (IDDM) or non-insulin dependent (NIDDM).

Ask about *symptoms*:

- presenting
  — weight loss, polyuria, polydipsia, dizziness, blurred vision, etc.

- of complications
  - e.g. pins and needles (peripheral neuropathy)
  - visual problems (? new vessel formation)
  - leg ulcers (infected feet)
  - vomiting
  - nocturnal diarrhoea
  - impotence
  - postural hypotension
  } autonomic neuropathy
  - intermittent claudication (peripheral vascular disease).

Signs

You are looking for the signs of the complications of diabetes.
Skin

- Necrobiosis lipoidica (yellow lesions on the shins, usually)
- Leg ulcers
- Infected feet/toes
- Injection sites (sometimes get fat atrophy which leaves skin hollowed out)
- Xanthelasmata (associated hyperlipidaemia)
- Granuloma annulare.

CVS

- Absent pulses in the lower limbs (peripheral vascular disease)
- Retinal changes
  - haemorrhages
  - exudates
  - new vessels
  - laser treatment
- Autonomic neuropathy (postural hypotension). This is confirmed by ECGs taken before, during and after a Valsalva manoeuvre and looking for changes in the R–R interval.

CNS

- Sensory ('glove and stocking') neuropathy
- Diabetic amyotrophy (femoral nerve damage causing wasting of quadriceps and absent knee jerk)
- Mononeuritis multiplex (multiple peripheral nerve palsies)
- Charcot's joints — painless, disorganised joint in a patient with a peripheral neuropathy.

Urogenital system. Signs of chronic renal failure (see p. 77). Make sure you ask to examine the urine. You will be looking for:

1. Glucose: ? compliance with treatment; ? correct level of treatment. Ask to look at a series of urine glucoses (or BM Stix).
2. Protein: microscopic albuminuria is the first sign of diabetic renal disease, and should be carefully screened for.
3. Ketones.

You need to know about the treatment and follow-up of diabetics. Spend a couple of sessions in the diabetic clinic if you have never been. The 'assessment and management of diabetic ketoacidosis' is a common written question and is not infrequently asked in the viva. Look these topics up in a standard text.

Causes of diabetes

- Idiopathic (95%)
- Steroid therapy, thiazide diuretics
- Pancreatitis, post-pancreatectomy
- Haemochromatosis
- Cushing's syndrome
- Acromegaly, phaeochromocytoma.

} rare

Hyperthyroidism

This is not a common case: most patients will be on, or have had, some form of treatment and will therefore (hopefully) be euthyroid. The diagnosis is usually given away by the typical facial appearance, with bulging eyes. However, the specific signs to look for are:

- agitation, sweating
- tremor (exaggerated physiological tremor)
- resting tachycardia
- atrial fibrillation
- exophthalmos
- lid lag/lid retraction
- goitre
- bruit over the thyroid
- pretibial myxoedema
- proximal myopathy.

} rare

Goitre

You may be asked to 'examine this patient's goitre'. Follow the simple scheme of:

1. look
2. feel
3. percuss (retrosternal goitre)
4. listen.

Look at the contours of the patient's neck from the front and the side. If it is a goitre there will be a swelling between the thyroid cartilage and the manubrium sterni. It may be mainly unilateral, particularly if there is a single nodule in the thyroid.

Now go behind the patient to palpate the thyroid with the flat of both hands (best done with the patient sitting in a chair). Ask the patient to have a sip from a glass of water and hold the water in her mouth. When you are ready, ask her to swallow whilst palpating the thyroid. If the swelling goes up on swallowing, the diagnosis is that of a goitre.

Now assess the characteristics of the goitre:

- smooth
  — Graves' disease
  — simple goitre (iodine-deficient)
  — multiple cysts
  — multinodular goitre
- single nodule
  — carcinoma of the thyroid
  — benign adenoma
  — single simple cyst
- tender
  — thyroiditis.

If you feel a single nodule, feel for local lymph nodes and attachment to local structures in the neck. These are features of a malignant thyroid nodule. Remember to listen for a bruit over the thyroid (ask the patient to hold her breath). This is sometimes heard in Graves' disease with a very vascular thyroid. You must now look for signs of hyper- or hypothyroidism.

Hypothyroidism

Again this is not a common examination case, for reasons given above.

Causes

- Idiopathic atrophy
- Post-[131] I therapy

- Post-thyroidectomy
- Post-Hashimoto's thyroiditis.

Signs

- Psychomotor retardation
- Dry scaly skin
- 'Peaches and cream' complexion
- Dry brittle hair, hair loss
- Loss of outer third of eyebrow (unreliable sign)
- Goitre
- Hoarse voice
- Weight gain
- Sinus bradycardia
- Carpal tunnel syndrome
- Slow-relaxing reflexes
- Cardiomyopathy
- Dementia   } rare
- Peripheral neuropathy
- Cerebellar degeneration.

Acromegaly

This is caused by a growth hormone-secreting adenoma in the pituitary gland. Even after treatment with bromocriptine or hypophysectomy (or both) the patient will still have residual signs of his disease. So, although acromegaly is a rare condition in everyday clinical practice, it is relatively common in the examination setting.

Signs

- Prominent jaw, nose, orbital ridges
- Large hands
- Large feet
- Typical facies
- Large, burly stature.

Remember to examine the visual fields for bitemporal hemianopia, which is caused by a local pressure effect of the tumour on the optic chiasm.

Complications of acromegaly

- Hypertension
- Proximal myopathy

- Carpal tunnel syndrome
- Osteoarthrosis (particularly of lower limbs)
- Cardiomyopathy (this is not infrequently the cause of death in the patient's 50s or 60s).

Associated conditions

- Diabetes
- Hypopituitarism
- Hypercalcaemia.

Cushing's syndrome

This syndrome is due to excess circulating corticosteroids.

Causes

(i)   Iatrogenic* — patients with conditions such as asthma or systemic lupus erythematosis are not infrequently treated with oral steroids and may exhibit some of the signs of Cushing's syndrome.

(ii) Cushing's disease — ACTH-secreting pituitary adenoma†.

(iii) Adrenal cortical adenoma.

(iv) Ectopic ACTH from bronchial carcinoma†.

The commonest cause, by far, is the iatrogenic variety.

Signs

- Moon face
- Fragile skin
- Easy bruising
- Buffalo hump
- Striae (abdominal wall)
- Hirsutism
- Muscular wasting
- Proximal myopathy.

Patients with Cushing's syndrome are more likely to develop diabetes, hypertension, recurrent infections and bone fractures (osteoporotic).

Note. Nelson's syndrome occurs after adrenalectomy for Cushing's disease. The main features are of pigmentation associated with the increase in circulating ACTH which follows such an operation.

Addison's disease[†]

In this condition there are insufficient circulating corticosteroids due to failure of the adrenal cortex. You will not see an untreated case in the exam. The patient may have been on treatment for many years and usually will have no clinical signs.

Causes

- Idiopathic* (autoimmune and associated with diabetes and thyroid disease)
- Metastatic deposits in the adrenal cortex from a primary in the lung or breast
- Tuberculosis[†] (calcified adrenals on plain abdominal X-ray).

Symptoms

- Weight loss
- Lassitude
- Postural hypotension
- Visual disturbance
- Vomiting.

Signs

- Pigmentation
  - hand (palmar creases)
  - knee
  - buccal
  - generalised
- Postural hypotension
- Fluid depletion.

The urea and electrolytes show hyponatraemia and hyperkalaemia.

Hypopituitarism[†]

Rare case.

Phaeochromocytoma[†]

Very rare exam case.

KEY QUESTIONS

ENDOCRINOLOGY

1. **What are the causes of:**
   - diabetes
   - goitre
   - Cushing's syndrome
   - Addison's disease?
2. **What clinical features suggest a malignant goitre?**
3. **Describe the more unusual ways in which the following diseases may present:**
   - diabetes
   - thyrotoxicosis
   - hypothyroidism
   - Addison's disease
   - Cushing's disease.
4. **What abnormalities are found in the serum glucose and urea and electrolytes in:**
   - Addison's disease
   - Cushing's disease?
5. **What are the clinical features of panhypopituitarism?**

3.7

Neurology

Neurological cases are regarded with some trepidation by many candidates. There are several reasons for this. Neurological disease can result in many signs, some of which carry rather long and unpronounceable names. A good neurological examination is an art form: when performed by an expert it can be a pleasure to watch. This is rarely the case in the examination room.

Candidates are sometimes wrong-footed by the question 'where is the lesion?'. Unfortunately, to give a meaningful answer you need to understand basic neuroanatomy: this raises the spectre of the dreaded (but long-forgotten) second MB. Before you start this chapter, therefore, I recommend you acquaint yourself with the following information from a standard anatomy textbook:

- sensory pathways
- motor pathways
- sensory dermatomes
- root values of:
  — peripheral nerves
  — muscle groups
  — reflex arcs
- gross anatomy of the brain, including brain stem, cranial nerves and their nuclei.

The most important thing to remember about a neurological examination is that it is *comparative*. In other words you test one sign on one side and then test on the other side and compare the difference. Do not forget to do this at all times: the examiners will be looking closely for it.

In the examination room you will never be asked to do a full neurological examination in the short cases — this would take far too long. Instead, the examiner will ask you to examine part of the nervous system (e.g. arms, legs, cranial nerves, cerebellum, etc.).

Table 3.7.1		
	UMN	LMN
Observation	—	Wasting, fasciculation
Tone	Spasticity	Hypotonicity
Power	Weakness	Weakness
Reflexes	Hyper-reflexia	Hyporeflexia
	Extensor plantars	
	Clonus	

You must be practised at doing such bits of a full neurological examination. It is for this reason that this chapter has been divided into the sections of 'regional neurology' as set out below:

- The head
  - eyes
  - cranial nerves
  - speech
  - higher functions
- Upper limb
- Lower limb
- Abnormal gait and movements
- Diffuse disease.

Many neurological problems will extend beyond the region you have been asked to examine. You must appreciate this and be seen to appreciate it by the examiners. For example, if you find ataxic nystagmus when asked to examine the eyes, you must be seen to look for other signs of multiple sclerosis.

Before you start the rest of the chapter it is important to appreciate the difference between upper motor neurone (UMN) and lower motor neurone (LMN) lesions. This is a frequently asked question (see Table 3.7.1).

Try to look stylish when you swing the patella hammer.

THE HEAD

EYES

Examination of the eyes causes mortal fear in some candidates. Actually this is unnecessary: eye cases are usually rather simple.

You need to have a good scheme for examination, a grasp of the essentials of using an ophthalmoscope and a knowledge of the cases which you are likely to meet.

Scheme for the examination of the eyes

Observation

Look at the patient's eyes at rest. The diagnosis may be obvious, e.g. exophthalmos (thyrotoxicosis), Horner's syndrome, etc. (see Fig. 3.7.1). Also look for xanthelasmata, senile arcus, etc.

Feel

Feel for increased tone in the eyes (palpation). This is a very inaccurate way of assessing intraocular pressure, which is normally measured by a very sensitive machine. Intraocular pressure is raised in conditions such as glaucoma.

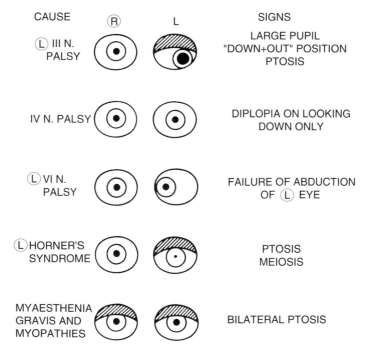

Fig. 3.7.1   Pupillary and eyelid abnormalities.

Visual acuity

Test this by asking the patient to read some small print (with glasses if he wears them), e.g. from a newspaper. A more formal assessment can be made with standard Snellen charts.

Visual fields

Sit on the edge of the patient's bed. Equilibrate the patient's visual fields with your own by making sure your heads are at the same level, 1 m apart. Ask the patient to cover one eye. Now cover your own eye (the opposite one to the one the patient has just covered). Test the patient's visual field (against your own) by slowly bringing a finger or white hat-pin from outside your field of vision (whilst the patient looks into your uncovered eye). Bring the hat-pin in at 2, 4, 8 and 10 o'clock, as this will pick up quadrantic field defects better. Now, using a red hat-pin, assess the blind spot (against your own) and look for scotomata (see common field defect, Fig. 3.7.2).

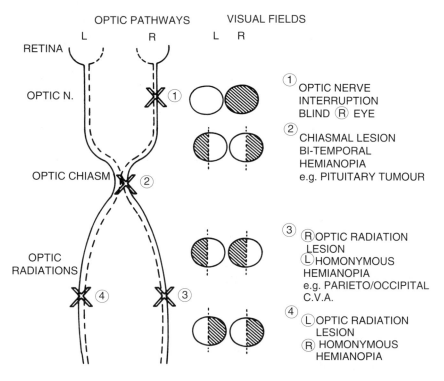

Fig. 3.7.2 Visual fields defects.

Fundoscopy

It is essential to be familiar with the ophthalmoscope you use during the examination. The only way to ensure that this happens is by taking either your own or one which you have borrowed. The patient should be in a darkened room with dilated pupils (ask for mydriatic drops if necessary). Set the machine with a plain lens and normal filters. Shine it onto your hand to check it is working. Now elicit the red reflex in both the patient's eyes. This is done by shining the light through the pupil from about 0.5 m. Light hits the retina and is reflected back as a red glow as you look through the lens of the ophthalmoscope. Anything which causes an interruption to this pathway of light will cause an absent red reflex, e.g:

- cataract
- prosthetic eye
- haemorrhage into anterior chamber
- vitreous haemorrhage.

Now examine the eye itself. Start off by asking the patient to look at a spot in the distance, ignoring the light of the ophthalmoscope. Approach the patient's eye from a slightly lateral direction. This approach has two advantages:

1. It enables the patient to concentrate on the spot in the distance, with minimal disturbance to his field of vision.
2. The optic disc should pop straight into view. (Focus on the optic disc by altering the lens strength to get a sharp image.) For short-sighted patients you will need a negative lens and for long-sighted patients you will need a positive lens. Once you have found the disc your problems should be over. Examine it carefully and assess:
    - colour
    - margin
    - contour.

If you cannot find the disc follow the vessels until it comes into view. Now look at all areas of the retina and in particular:

- vessels
    — tortuosity
    — silver wiring
    — a-v nipping
    — new vessel formation
    — haemorrhages.

- retinal surface
  — haemorrhages
  — exudates
  — evidence of laser therapy.

Now slowly 'rack back' by increasing the lens strength of the ophthalmoscope. Check the posterior chamber, lens (for cataracts) and anterior chamber. With practice fundoscopy will become easier. Examine as many normal fundi as possible. Remember that negroid and Asian retinae look much darker than caucasian ones.

Move

You will be essentially testing cranial nerves III, IV and VI and the intraocular muscles which they supply. Stand to the left of the patient. Rest your left hand on the patient's forehead (to help keep it still). Now, asking the patient to follow the index finger of your right hand, test all directions of movement. Ask the patient to say 'yes' if he sees double. Try to find out in which direction of gaze the double vision is worst. Look for:

- failure of gaze (and direction)
- nystagmus
- dysconjugate gaze.

Note: make sure you do not confuse physiological and pathological nystagmus. To avoid this mistake remember the following two tips:

1. do not draw the patient's gaze too far laterally
2. do not place the finger too close to the patient's eyes (0.5 m is usually ideal).

TYPICAL CASES

NEUROLOGY — EYES

- Fundoscopy
- Ptosis
- Horner's syndrome
- Large pupil
- Small pupil
- Nystagmus

Fundoscopy

Normal appearance of fundus

It would be a bit naughty of the examiner to give you a normal fundus (see Fig. 3.7.3). However, until you know what is or isn't normal, fundoscopy will prove difficult.

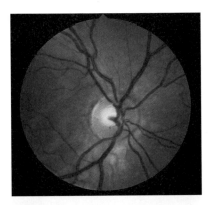

Fig. 3.7.3   Normal fundus.

Optic atrophy

If the disc looks surprisingly white, distinct and much easier to find than normal, it is probably optic atrophy (Fig. 3.7.4). It is absolutely essential to compare it with the disc on the other side.

Causes

- Multiple sclerosis

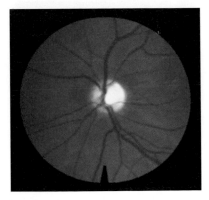

Fig. 3.7.4   Optic atrophy.

- Post-traumatic
- Retro-orbital tumour
- Diabetes
- Retinal artery thrombosis.

Proliferative diabetic retinopathy

The reason new vessels occur in the diabetic fundus is due to retinal ischaemia. It is important to recognise NVD (Fig. 3.7.5) as untreated such patients rapidly go blind. Figure 3.7.6 shows the condition with new vessels elsewhere (NVE).

Other signs commonly seen in the diabetic eye include:

- haemorrhages
- exudates
- cataracts.

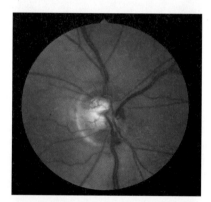

Fig. 3.7.5 Proliferative diabetic retinopathy with new vessels on disc (NVD).

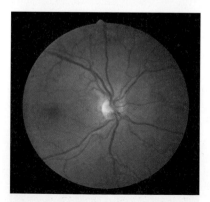

Fig. 3.7.6 Proliferative diabetic retinopathy with new vessels elsewhere (NVE).

Severe hypertensive retinopathy with papilloedema

Hypertensive retinopathy is classified as severe if papilloedema is present. Severe hypertensive retinopathy is usually seen in young or middle-aged patients with accelerated hypertension, often of renal origin (e.g. glomerulonephritis). Figure 3.7.7 shows some of the other changes seen in the fundus in hypertensives including arteriolar narrowing, hard and soft exudates.

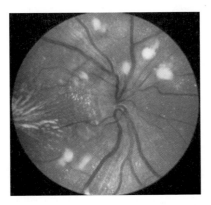

Fig. 3.7.7   Severe hypertensive retinopathy with papilloedema.

Causes (of papilloedema)

• Accelerated hypertension
• Benign intracranial hypertension
• Raised intracranial pressure (any cause).

Hint.   If you find the disc difficult or impossible to find, papilloedema is probably present.

Retinitis pigmentosa

Figure 3.7.8 shows the classical 'bone spicule' appearance around the periphery of the retina. The purple spot at the fovea is artefactual (caused by the light reflex when the photograph was taken).

Retinitis pigmentosa is a genetic disorder and may be autosomal dominant, autosomal recessive or X-linked. As the peripheral part of the retina is affected first, patients may present with night blindness and tunnel vision. Central vision acuity is relatively spared in the early stages of the disease. Most patients are registered blind

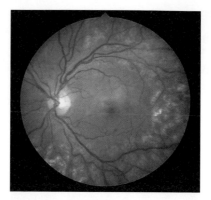

Fig. 3.7.8 Retinitis pigmentosa.

by their 30s, although this is variable and depends to some extent on the genetic type.

Glass eye

Some nasty examiners will ask you to perform fundoscopy on a prosthetic eye (Fig. 3.7.9). If you remember to do the red reflex first you will stay one step ahead.

Fig. 3.7.9 Fundoscopic appearance of a glass eye.

Ptosis (drooping of the eyelid)

Causes

- Third nerve palsy (large pupil)
- Part of Horner's syndrome (small pupil)

- Myopathies (usually bilateral ptosis)
  — myaesthenia gravis
  — myotonia congenita
  — other congenital myopathies, e.g. facio/scapulo humeral
    idiopathic.

  Note. Bilateral ptosis, particularly if mild, can be difficult to spot.

Horner's syndrome

This is rare in practice, but common in exams. There is a classical combination of signs, which is:

- ptosis
- enophthalmos
- meiosis (small pupil)
- ipsilateral loss of sweating (face).

It is caused by interruption of the sympathetic supply to levator palpebrae superioris and dilator pupillae. This can be caused by lesions in the brain stem, stellate ganglion or root of neck.

Causes

- Carcinoma of bronchus (Pancoast tumour)
- Syringomyelia (UMN signs in legs, LMN signs in arms)
- Syringobulbia (bulbar palsy)
- Sympathectomy
- Tumour at root of neck, cervical cord.

Large pupil

Causes

- Mydriatic drops*
- Holmes–Adie pupil* (dilated pupil, which responds very slowly to light plus absent ankle jerks in young females)
- Third nerve palsy
- Surgical (irregular pupil) iridectomy, cataract removal.

Small pupil

Causes

- Old age*
- Horner's syndrome

- Pilocarpine (treatment for glaucoma)
- Argyll Robertson pupil[†] (irregular pupil) with absent light reflex found in syphilis.

Nystagmus

Describe it in terms of the fast phase of movement.

Horizontal nystagmus — causes

- Vestibular causes (associated with deafness and vertigo)
  — Meniere's disease
  — middle ear surgery
  — multiple sclerosis
  — syringobulbia
  — viral labyrinthitis.
- Cerebellar causes (look for other cerebellar signs)
  — tumour, primary or secondary
  — degenerative disease
  — multiple sclerosis
  — cerebrovascular disease.

THE CRANIAL NERVES

The examiners may ask you to examine the whole lot, but more often they will select a single cranial nerve for you to examine. This is most often the VIIth cranial nerve (see Table 3.7.2).

Scheme for examining the cranial nerves

II

- Acuity
- Visual fields   } See pp 90–92
- Fundoscopy.

III, IV, VI (see p. 92)

VII*

Test the facial muscles:

Table 3.7.2 Cranial nerve palsies

Cranial nerve	Sign	Causes
I[†]	Smell (bottles)	Frontal lobe tumour Fractured skull
II	Visual fields • scotomata • field loss (Fig. 3.7.2) Fundoscopy • papillitis • optic atrophy Pupillar reflexes • visual acuity	MS Retro-orbital tumour Alcohol Tobacco Macular degeneration
III	Ptosis, large pupil, eye deviation (down and out)	Cavemous sinus thrombosis Raised intracranial pressure
IV[†]	Diplopia on downward gaze	
VI	Failure of lateral gaze (Fig. 3.7.1)	
V[†] motor	Jaw deviates to side of lesion	Cerebello–pontine angle tumour
sensory	Anaesthetic area (depends on branch affected) reduced corneal reflex (V^1)	
VII*	Ipsilateral face drop Bell's sign (LMN only)	Idiopathic (Bell's palsy) Middle ear • tumour • infection Post-surgical Sarcoid (sometimes bilateral)
VIII[†]	Weber and Rinne tests (see notes)	Wax ⎫ Otitis media ⎬ Conductive Otosclerosis ⎭ deafness Trauma ⎫ Infection ⎪ Perceptive VIII nerve ⎬ deafness tumour ⎪ (sensorineural) Streptomycin ⎭
IX ⎫ X ⎭	Uvula deviates away from affected side	*Unilateral lesion* Tumour or deposits around jugular foramen
XI	Reduced bulk of trapezius Reduced power on shrugging shoulders and sternocleidomastoid	
XII	Ipsilateral wasting of tongue Deviation of tongue to affected side Tongue fasciculation	*Bilateral lesions* Syringobulbia Motor neurone disease (MND)

Notes to Table 3.7.2

1. When examining the VII nerve: if you think it is an LMN lesion, always look behind the ipsilateral ear and over the ipsilateral parotid for scars (mastoid and parotid surgery respectively). These are common causes of this problem, and will make your examination look classy.
2. Look for Bell's sign (LMN VIIth). On attempted eye closure the ipsilateral eye deviates upwards.
3. The following can cause any cranial nerve lesion:
   - diabetes
   - multiple sclerosis (MS)
   - sarcoid
   - nerve tumour
   - post-meningitis.
4. *Rinne's test.* Hold a tuning fork on the mastoid process until it is no longer audible. Now hold it by the external auditory canal: in the normal ear it should now be audible (air conduction [AC] > bone conduction [BC]). In perceptive deafness (VIIIth nerve problem) this situation persists. In conductive deafness BC > AC because air-conducted sound depends on intact auditory ossicles for its transmission.
5. *Weber's test.* Place a tuning fork on the vertex of the skull. In normal people it is heard equally well in both ears. In sensory deafness the tuning fork will not be heard in the affected ear. In conductive deafness, the noise will be heard equally well in both ears. This is because the auditory ossicles are bypassed by direct bone conduction.
   - Orbicularis oculi ('screw your eyes up tight and don't let me open them').
   - Orbicularis ori ('smile, keep your lips together and don't let me open them').
   - Frontalis muscle ('raise your eyebrows').

This last test distinguishes an upper motor neurone (UMN) VIIth from a lower motor neurone (LMN) VIIth lesion. In the latter there is total 'face drop', including frontalis (forehead). In a UMN VIIth nerve lesion the forehead is spared, because of bilateral cortical representation of the frontalis muscle. This is a very commonly asked question.

Summary.   UMN VII forehead spared, LMN VII total face drop.

Examination of the other cranial nerves is summarised in Table 3.7.2.

SPEECH

Dysarthria

This is a difficulty in the physical articulation of the spoken word caused by a failure of the elements of the speech 'end organ' (i.e. a local cause). There are degrees of dysarthria, and mild dysarthria can be made more pronounced by one of the standard tongue-twisters: 'West Register Street'; 'baby hippopotamus'.

Causes

- Ill-fitting dentures*
- Cranial nerve palsy VII, IX, X, XII
- Bulbar palsy
- Pseudobulbar palsy ('hot potato' speech)
- Cerebellar disease ('staccato' speech).

Bulbar palsy is caused by bilateral LMN lesions of cranial nerves IX, X, XII. Patients often complain of nasal regurgitation. Signs include fasciculating tongue and loss of gag reflex. It is rare and usually caused by motor neurone disease.

Pseudobulbar palsy is caused by bilateral UMN lesions (e.g. bilateral CVAs). It is more common than a true bulbar palsy. Patients complain of nasal regurgitation and relatives may say that the patient cries inappropriately (labile emotions). They have a characteristic speech which is high-pitched but rather nasal ('hot potato' or 'Donald Duck' speech). In addition they have a positive jaw jerk and may have bilateral UMN signs in the limbs.

Dysphasia

There are two types of dysphasia, expressive (or nominal) and receptive.

In *expressive dysphasia*, which is due to a lesion in Broca's motor speech area (fronto-parietal), there is a failure of speech content or expression. This results in the patient being unable to name familiar objects such as a pen, jacket, etc., whilst knowing what they are. Its usual cause is a CVA in the dominant hemisphere.

Receptive dysphasia is due to failure of integration of hearing and speech. This results in the patient being unable to understand the spoken word. It is usually caused by a CVA or other lesion in Wernicke's area of the dominant hemisphere (temporo/parietal).

Aphasia is the inability to speak at all.

Patients with both expressive and receptive dysphasia will be unable to name familiar objects. The way to quickly distinguish the two types of dysphasia is as follows:

Q. 'Can you tell me what this is?' (show the patient a pen).
   Neither will give a meaningful reply.
Q. 'Is it a watch?'
   Receptive dysphasic: no meaningful reply.
   Expressive dysphasic: 'No!'
Q. 'Is it a key?'
   Receptive dysphasic: no meaningful reply.
   Expressive dysphasic: 'No!'
Q. 'Is it a pen?'
   Receptive dysphasic: no meaningful reply.
   Expressive dysphasic: 'Yes?'

HIGHER FUNCTIONS

General cerebral function

Patients with a generalised systemic disease or generalised disease of cerebral substance often have intellectual impairment. You ought to have a list of questions at your fingertips to demonstrate such problems:

— name
— age
— address
— date of birth
— name of monarch
— name of prime minister
— dates of Second World War
— time
— recent newsworthy events
— day of week
— date
— place of interview?

Additional tests such as ability to remember three objects, ability to serially subtract 7 from 100 and ability to remember a six figure number can also be valuable. Personally, I have found the name of the current prime minister to be a most valuable question: patients who get this wrong tend to have a very severe cerebral dysfunction.

Frontal lobe function[†]

Patients with frontal lobe problems tend to be disinhibited. They may wander. They are frequently incontinent. Valuable information is gained from relatives/neighbours.

Parietal lobe function[†]

On a superficial examination there may be no abnormalities, unless specifically looked for:

- sensory inattention (non-dominant hemisphere)
- apraxia (loss of fine movements associated with a complicated task, e.g. dressing, retrieving a match from a closed matchbox)
- astereognosis (inability to recognise object placed in hand with eyes closed)
- dyslexia (reading difficulties)
- dysgraphia (writing difficulties)
- dyscalculia (mathematical difficulties)
- left/right disorientation
- finger agnosia (inability to recognise objects by touch).

THE UPPER LIMB

Scheme for the examination of the upper limb

Observation

- Wasting   ⎫
- Fasciculation ⎬ LMN lesions
- Posture, e.g. 'waiter's tip', 'claw hand'
- Scars, e.g. ulnar nerve transposition.

Tone

- Increased (UMN)
- Decreased (LMN)
- Cogwheel (extrapyramidal).

Power

Root values	Movement
C3, 4	Shoulder abduction
C5, 6	Shoulder adduction
	Elbow flexion
C7	Elbow ⎫
	Wrist ⎬ Extension
	Finger ⎭
C8, T1	Small muscles of hand

Peripheral nerve motor supply

- Ulnar: all small muscles of hand with the exception of 'LOAF' (median nerve) muscles
- Median
  — **L**ateral two lumbricals (flexion of M/P joints)
  — **O**pponens pollicis
  — **A**bductor pollicis
  — **F**lexor pollicis brevis
- Radial: wrist and finger extensors.

Sensation

Test:
- pain (pinprick)
- light touch (cotton wool)
- joint position sense
- vibration (tuning fork).

Temperature sensation is usually irrelevant in the exam.

You must map out the area of sensory loss and try to deduce whether it is a root or peripheral nerve problem. Remember to compare the sides (see Figs 3.7.10 and 3.7.11 for sensory supply of upper limb).

Reflexes

Reflex	Root
Biceps	C5, 6
Supinator	C6
Triceps	C7, 8

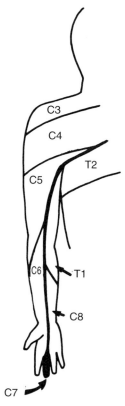

Fig. 3.7.10   Sensory dermatomes: upper limbs. C7 is the key to working it out; this supplies middle finger of hand. Note the C4/T2 interface on the upper chest wall.

Cerebellar signs

- Past pointing
- Intention tremor
- Dysdiadochokinesis.

Involuntary movements

- Tremor
- Athetosis
- Chorea
- Ballismus.

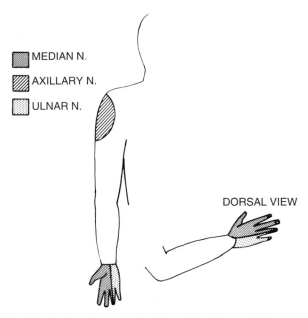

Fig. 3.7.11   Distribution of sensory loss in peripheral nerve lesions: upper limbs. NB: radial nerve palsies often result in no demonstrable sensory loss (overlapping nerve supply). Patients sometimes complain of paraesthesiae over dorsum of thumb.

TYPICAL CASES

NEUROLOGY — THE UPPER LIMB

- The wasted hand
- Ulnar nerve palsy
- Median nerve palsy
- Radial nerve palsy
- Nerve to serratus anterior
- C5, C6 root
- T1 root (Klumpke's palsy)
- UMN signs
- LMN signs
- Sensory problems
- Proximal myopathy
- Parkinson's syndrome
- Cerebellar signs

The wasted hand*

Very common case. There are many causes of wasting of the small muscles of the hand:

- non-neurological
  - old age★
  - rheumatoid arthritis★
- neurological
  - cervical rib
  - T1 root lesion
  - ulnar nerve palsy
  - syringomyelia   } Often
  - motor neurone disease. } bilateral signs

Try to ascertain the cause. Remember that MND and syringomyelia may have UMN signs in the legs. Look for scars around the elbow (ulnar nerve palsy). It can be difficult to sort out whether it is a T1 root lesion or an ulnar palsy. Table 3.7.3 will help.

Ulnar nerve palsy

Usually at the elbow (often traumatic) (see Table 3.7.3).

Table 3.7.3 Ulnar nerve and T1 root palsies		
	Power	Sensory loss
T1 root	Reduced in all small muscles of hand	Often little
Ulnar nerve	LOAF not affected (median nerve supply)	Inner aspect of medial $1\frac{1}{2}$ fingers and inner aspect of forearm

Median nerve palsy*

Very common. It will usually be due to carpal tunnel syndrome.

Signs

- Reduced power in LOAF
- Sensory loss lateral $3\frac{1}{2}$ fingers
- Tinel's sign (tapping over median nerve at the wrist causes paraesthesiae).

Causes of carpal tunnel syndrome

- Myxoedema
- Acromegaly
- Rheumatoid arthritis
- Pregnancy
- Trauma.

It is most common in middle-aged women with none of the above.

Radial nerve palsy[†]

Wrist drop due to radial nerve palsy (usually) as it passes through the spiral groove. Finger extension and elbow extension are also reduced. It is common in alcoholics and this is the reason for it also being known as 'Saturday night palsy'. After a Saturday night binge, the patient falls sound asleep in the armchair whilst watching TV, his arms having flopped over the edge of the chair. In this position the radial nerve (in the spiral groove) is exposed to trauma from the arm of the chair. Next morning, on awakening, the arm is fairly useless (try to use your own fingers with your wrist fully flexed!), but usually recovers spontaneously.

Nerve to serratus anterior (C5, 6, 7)[†]

Causes 'winging of the scapula'.

C5, C6 root (Erb–Duchenne palsy)

Causes

- Birth trauma
- Falling from a motorbike onto the tip of the shoulder.

Signs

- Posture — 'waiter tip sign' (the arm is held internally rotated with flexion of the metacarpophalangeal joints)
- Reduced sensation on outer aspect of the arm
- Absent biceps and supinator jerks
- C5, 6 motor loss (see earlier).

T1 root (Klumpke's palsy)

Causes
- Birth trauma
- Trauma
- Cervical rib
- Pancoast tumour.

Signs
- Wasted hand (clawed)
- Sensory loss on inner aspect of upper arm.

UMN signs

- Unilateral
  — e.g. CVA
  — cerebral tumour
- Bilateral
  — e.g. bilateral CVAs
  — MS
  — high cord lesion
  — syringobulbia
  — motor neurone disease (often LMN signs predominate in upper limbs).

LMN signs

- Unilateral* (see first seven cases)
- Bilateral
  — syringomyelia
  — MND
  — bilateral cervical ribs.

Sensory problems[†]

Sensory signs are usually found in conjunction with motor signs, as already outlined. It is extremely rare to get a peripheral sensory neuropathy which solely affects the hands: symptoms in the lower limbs usually predominate.

Proximal myopathy[†]

Weakness of proximal muscles. Patients find difficulty in raising their arms (e.g. combing the hair).

Causes

- Polymyositis
- Dermatomyositis — heliotrope rash under eyes/erythematous rash over hands (50% have an underlying carcinoma)
- Cushing's syndrome
- Thyrotoxicosis
- Carcinoma
- Diabetes
- Hereditary.

Don't forget to check the power in the proximal muscles of the legs as these are often affected (inability to stand from the sitting position with the arms folded across the chest).

Parkinson's syndrome (see pp 116–117)

Cerebellar signs (see pp 117–118)

THE LOWER LIMB

Scheme for examination of the lower limb

Use the same routine as that for the upper limb.

Inspection

- Wasting
- Scars
- Foot drop, etc.

Tone

Power

Root	Muscle group
L1, 2	Hip flexion
L3, 4	Knee extension
L5, S1	Knee flexion
L4, L5	Ankle dorsiflexion
S1	Ankle plantar flexion

Reflexes

- Knee — L3, 4
- Ankle — L5, S1.

Knee and ankle clonus are found in upper motor neurone lesions.

Sensory assessment (see Fig. 3.7.12)

Remember that sensory dermatomes in the lower limb are rather less clearcut than in the upper limbs.

Coordination

- Heel/shin test.

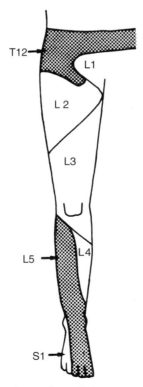

Fig. 3.7.12   Sensory dermatomes: lower limbs.

Romberg's test

Ask the patient to close her eyes whilst standing. Romberg's test is positive if the patient now falls over. It is a test of dorsal column function.

Gait (see pp 115–117)

TYPICAL CASES

NEUROLOGY — THE LOWER LIMB

- Sensory neuropathy
- Foot drop
- Root lesions
- Unilateral UMN signs
- Bilateral UMN signs
- Hereditary sensory motor neuropathies

Sensory neuropathy*

Common case. Symmetrical sensation loss. All modalities affected. 'Glove and stocking' distribution, but lower limbs affected first and more severely.

Causes

- Alcohol*
- Diabetes*
- Carcinomatosis*
- Drugs (e.g. nitrofurantoin)
- Vitamin deficiency (especially the B group).

Rare causes: Guillan–Barre syndrome, amyloid, sarcoid, uraemia, myeloma, porphyria, leprosy.

Remember to look for the consequences of neuropathy, e.g.

- painless ulcers
- Charcot's joints (ankle, knee).

Foot drop

Lateral peroneal nerve palsy. It is often caused by trauma to the head of the fibula (bumper-bar injury) but can be found spontaneously in diabetics.

Signs

- Foot drop
- High stepping gait on affected side
- Sensory examination } Normal
- Reflexes. } Normal

Other causes of foot drop

- Mononeuritis multiplex
- Peripheral neuropathy
- Motor neurone disease
- Peroneal muscular atrophy (Charcot–Marie–Tooth syndrome).

Root lesions[†]

L5

- Weakness of extensors of the great toe
- Reduced/absent ankle jerk
- Reduced sensation over L5 dermatome.

S1

- Reduced power
  — plantar flexion
  — foot eversion
- Absent ankle jerk
- Reduced sensation over outer aspect of foot.

L2–4

These root lesions are very rare. They are caused by:

- prolapsed intervertebral disc*
- metastases
- meningioma.

Unilateral UMN signs*

Found in common-or-garden cerebrovascular accidents.

Bilateral UMN signs (spastic paraparesis)

Rare in practice, common in examinations.

Signs

- Bilateral
  — hypertonia
  — hyper-reflexia
  — plantar extensors
  — ankle/knee clonus
  — weakness
  — sensory loss.

You *must* look for a 'sensory level' (use a pin on abdominal and thoracic walls). This will tell you the level of the lesion in the spinal cord.

Causes

- Trauma (usually RTA)
- Vertebral collapse
  — metastatic cancer
  — osteoporosis
- Tumours
  — extradural
    — meningioma
    — angioma
    — neurofibroma
    — metastases
  — intrinsic, e.g. glioma
- Spinal artery embolism
- Multiple sclerosis
- Motor neurone disease
- Syringomyelia/bulbia.

Hereditary sensory motor neuropathies[†]

Peroneal muscular atrophy. Types I and II used to be known as 'Charcot–Marie–Tooth' disease.

Rare case. Autosomal dominant condition causing wasting of peroneal muscles in early adult life. Eventually all the lower leg muscles waste, causing the 'inverted champagne bottle' appearance.

Signs

- Wasting
- Foot drop
- Impaired vibration sense and general sensory loss
- Signs in the upper limbs (very rare).

ABNORMAL GAIT AND MOVEMENTS

ABNORMAL GAIT

Cerebrovascular accident (CVA)*

There is a rigid leg and partially plantar flexed foot. The patient drags his leg through a semicircle.

Spastic paraplegia

The patient drags both spastic legs. He usually swings the upper torso to help him move. This has been described as a 'wading through mud gait'.

Dorsal column loss

The patient looks at the ground. He has a wide-based gait with high foot lift. The patient will fall if the eyes are closed (Romberg's sign). The patient may also have loss of joint position and vibration sense.

Causes

- Diabetes
- Friedreich's ataxia
- Subacute combined degeneration of the cord } rare
- Tabes dorsalis.

ᴐp gait

ᴣ stepping gait. Feet slap the ground.

Causes

- Lateral peroneal nerve palsy
- Poliomyelitis
- Charcot–Marie–Tooth disease
- Motor neurone disease.

Proximal myopathy

Waddling gait (looks like a duck). The upper torso swings to aid forward propulsion of the limbs. The patient will have difficulty getting out of a chair (see pp 109–110).

Parkinson's disease*

Shuffling gait. Small steps. The patient is stooped and rigid, and finds turning difficult. The arms do not swing. Festination (sudden increase in speed of walking). On/off phenomenon (patient suddenly 'freezes' during a movement — a most distressing symptom). Patients with Parkinson's disease find initiating movements difficult. Remember to assess how the patient's illness affects his daily life, e.g dressing (buttons may be impossible), eating, etc.

Other signs

- Tremor
  - 6 Hz
  - pill rolling
  - better during voluntary action
- Bradykinesia
  - facial immobility
- Rigidity (cogwheel).

Causes

- Idiopathic
- Drugs, e.g. major tranquillisers

- Drug abuse, e.g. MTPT
- Vascular (multiple CVAs to the basal ganglia). This variety is usually unresponsive to therapy
- Post-viral (encephalitis lethargia occurred in the early 1920s — most of these patients are now dead).
- Repeated trauma, e.g. boxers.

Cerebellar disease

Veering gait. Patients fall to side of the lesion (this is accentuated by asking the patient to walk along an imaginary white line on the floor).

Other signs (all ipsilateral)

- Dysarthria
- Nystagmus (fast phase to side of lesion)
- Intention tremor (this is an oscillating tremor which is worse on movement)
- Past pointing (finger–nose test)
- Dysdiadochokinesis
- Poor heel/shin test
- Cerebellar drift (when the patient holds his hands outstretched there is ipsilateral upward drift or oscillation)
- Hypotonia
- Hyporeflexia.

Causes

- CVA*
  — haemorrhage
  — infarction
- Tumour
  — secondary*
  — primary
  — non-metastatic degeneration (with carcinoma of the bronchus)
- Degenerative
  — multiple sclerosis
  — alcoholism
  — familial, e.g. Friedreich's ataxia
  — hypothyroidism[†].

Note. Lesions of the cerebellar vermis (central part of the cerebellum) cause a peculiar sign called truncal ataxia. This results in instability and writhing movements of the upper torso, accentuated by asking the patient to sit forwards with his arms folded.

ABNORMAL MOVEMENTS

Tremor

Resting

- Physiological* (worse with alcohol)
- Parkinson's disease*
- Benign essential tremor (better with alcohol, often familial)
- Wilson's disease.

Note. Treatment with β_2 agonists and thyrotoxicosis cause an exaggerated physiological tremor.

Worse on movement

- Cerebellar tremor (intention tremor).

Note. Severe Parkinsonian and benign essential tremors are sometimes worse on movement.

Chorea

Sudden, rapid involuntary and purposeless jerks or fragments of movements. The patient appears fidgety. It is usually a sign of extrapyramidal disease.

Causes

- Drugs, e.g. L-dopa
- CVA (basal ganglia)
- Tumour (basal ganglia)
- Sydenham's chorea
- Thyrotoxicosis
- SLE.

Athetosis

Slow, writhing, sinuous movements. Extrapyramidal.

Causes

- Cerebral palsy*
- Post-cerebral anoxia (e.g. cardiac arrest, drowning, etc.)
- Wilson's disease
- Hereditary.

Hemiballismus[†]

Wild flinging movements in upper limb, due to an ipsilateral lesion to subthalamic nucleus. Responds to chlorpromazine.

DIFFUSE NEUROLOGICAL DISEASE

Many neurological diseases cut across artificial anatomical boundaries. Be prepared to ask to examine other aspects of the nervous system, if you think this is relevant.

CVA*

This causes a pyramidal weakness in both the upper and lower limbs, if the lesion involves the cerebral cortex, internal capsule, or pyramidal tracts as they run through the brain stem. It is important to know the classical distribution of a pyramidal motor weakness.

The weak muscle groups are:

- shoulder abduction
- elbow and wrist extension
- finger abduction
- hip flexors
- hamstrings
- dorsiflexion of foot.

The easy way to remember this is to recall the typical posture of a stroke victim, due to the stronger, intact (spastic) muscle groups. The arm is adducted at the shoulder and flexed at the elbow and wrist. The leg is held straight and the foot drags on walking, due to intact glutei, quadriceps and plantar flexors.

If you find a pyramidal weakness in one leg it is important to examine the ipsilateral arm and controlateral leg for signs of pyramidal weakness. This is because the causes of a spastic hemiparesis and a spastic paraparesis are quite different (see p. 114).

Multiple sclerosis*

This is a diffuse demyelinating process of unknown aetiology. It commonly starts in early adult life and affects women more frequently than men. It seems to be more common in temperate zones. Spontaneous relapses and remissions occur, but there is usually a gradual overall deterioration through the years. Patients commonly end up wheelchair-bound in the later stages of the disease. The signs will depend on the sites involved and the stage of the disease:

- UMN deficit
  - — hemiparesis
  - — paraparesis
  - — monoparesis
- cerebellar signs
  - — often bilateral
  - — ataxic nystagmus (pathognomonic)
- optic atrophy
- sensory disturbances
- III, IV or VI nerve palsies
- painless retention of urine
- cerebral cortex involvement — inappropriate euphoria is frequently seen in the later stages of the disease, due to frontal lobe demyelination.

Motor neurone disease

Exceptionally rare in clinical practice. Not quite so rare in exams. There is a progressive, idiopathic degeneration of the anterior horn cells (spinal cord), cranial nerve nuclei and pyramidal tracts. There are *no* sensory signs. There are three patterns of neurological signs, but there is often overlap between these groups:

1. *True bulbar palsy* (see p. 101) — bilateral cranial nerve palsies of IX–XII.
2. *Progressive muscular atrophy* — bilateral degeneration of the anterior horn cells. This causes bilateral lower motor neurone signs in the hands, followed by the feet. There is prominent muscle fasciculation. Loss of deep tendon reflexes.
3. *Amyotrophic lateral sclerosis* — pyramidal tract degeneration; spastic paraparesis. Arms are usually affected later (and less extensively).

Syringomyelia[†]

Cyst in cervical spinal cord (anterior position). It presents in early adult life and slowly progresses over 20 years. The cyst encroaches on tracts which lie anteriorly:

- lateral spinothalamic (pain and temperature)
- anterior horn cells (LMN)
- pyramidal (UMN).

Signs

- Dissociated sensory loss (arms)
- Painless lesions in the upper limbs
- Charcot's joints (wrist, elbow)
- Wasting of the small muscles of the hand
- UMN signs in the legs.

Syringobulbia[†]

Same as syringomyelia, but the lesion is in the lower brain stem/ upper cervical cord. The signs are very similar, but in addition there may be:

- ipsilateral V nerve palsy ⎱ Involvement of cranial
- bulbar palsy ⎰ nerve nuclei
- ipsilateral Horner's syndrome (cervical sympathetic nerves)
- nystagmus (brain stem cerebellar connections).

KEY QUESTIONS

NEUROLOGY

1. What are the causes of:
   - ptosis
   - VI nerve palsy
   - XII nerve palsy
   - pseudobulbar palsy
   - anosmia
   - wasting of the hand
   - carpal tunnel syndrome
   - proximal myopathy
   - parkinsonism
   - sensory neuropathy
   - spastic paraparesis
   - dorsal column loss
   - cerebellar disease
   - resting tremor?
2. **Which muscles of the hand are served by the median nerve?**
3. **What are the causes of an absent red reflex?**
4. **What is Romberg's sign? What is its significance?**
5. **What are the neurological manifestations of the acquired immune-deficiency syndrome?**
6. **What is the difference, on clinical examination, between an ulnar nerve palsy and a T1 root lesion?**

3.8

Rheumatology

Rheumatological cases are common in Final MB because rheumatological disease is common, often resulting in chronic physical signs.

Scheme for examination of the joints

Look — Feel — Move

Inspection

General. Start by observing the patient generally. Active attention to this point may give you the diagnosis immediately, e.g.:

- butterfly rash on face (SLE)
- small mouth, beaked nosed (scleroderma)
- stooped posture (ankylosing spondylitis)
- scaly rash (psoriatic arthropathy).

Joints. Now concentrate on the joint(s) in question. The examiner will tell you which joint(s) he wishes you to examine. Look at the joints from the front, back and sides. In particular you are looking for:

- swelling
- erythema
- joint deformity
- scars (previous surgery).

Palpation

Always ask the patient if the joint(s) are tender — if they are, you must palpate carefully. Try not to hurt the patient (keep glancing at her face). Look for:

- tenderness
- synovial thickening
- joint effusion
- deformity
- associated muscle wasting.

Movement

Passive. Move the patient's joint (gently) to assess its range in all directions of normal movement. Again, be careful, it is easy to hurt the patient.

Active. Now ask the patient to move the joint herself in the same modalities.

Functional movement. Try to get an idea of how the patient's joint disease has affected that joint's function, e.g.:

- hip joint
  — ask the patient to walk, stand from the sitting position
- hand
  — grip
  — thumb opposition
  — writing
  — use of knife and fork
  — buttoning a shirt, etc.

Further aspects of examination

As directed by your findings. *Always* look for rheumatoid nodules on the elbows. Also look for:

- nail changes ⎱ psoriatic
- skin lesions ⎰ arthropathy
- gouty tophi (ear, periarticular)
- scleroderma facies/skin
- nailfold telangiectasia (SLE, RA)
- butterfly rash (SLE).

TYPICAL CASES

RHEUMATOLOGY

- Rheumatoid arthritis
- Systemic lupus erythematosus
- Scleroderma
- Ankylosing spondylitis
- Psoriatic arthropathy
- Monoarthritis
- Raynaud's phenomenon

Rheumatoid arthritis (RA)*

Most commonly you are presented with a pair of arthritic hands. Often, with end-stage disease, the diagnosis is obvious. Occasionally you are presented with more acute joints. This is more difficult. The diagnosis may not be immediately obvious, and there is a risk of hurting the patient. If the skin overlying a joint is erythematous proceed with caution.

Signs

- Hands
  — swelling
  — erythema
  — synovial thickening/tenderness
  — wasting of the small muscles of the hand
  — deformity, e.g. metacarpophalangeal subluxation
  — ulnar deviation
  — swan neck deformity ⎫
  — Boutonniere deformity ⎬ See Fig. 3.8.1
  — 'Z' deformity of the thumb ⎭
  — reduced function
- Always look for rheumatoid nodules (Figs 3.8.2 and 3.8.3)
- Ask about other affected joints.

Rheumatoid arthritis usually, but not always, affects joints symmetrically. In the hand the proximal joints, e.g. the metacarpophalangeal joints (MCP) and the proximal interphalangeal

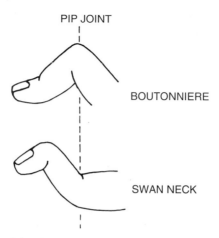

PIP JOINT

BOUTONNIERE

SWAN NECK

Fig. 3.8.1 Finger deformities: rheumatoid arthritis.

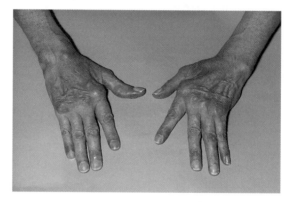

Fig. 3.8.2 Rheumatoid arthritis. Note the prominent metacarpal heads (metacarpophalangeal subluxation), ulnar deviation of the fingers and wasting of the small muscles of the hand.

(PIP) joints are predominantly affected. RA is much more common in females.

Complications of RA

RA is a systemic disease and the complications include:

- Sjögren's syndrome
  — dry eyes
  — dry mouth
  — arthritis

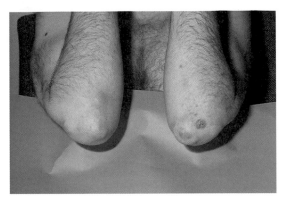

Fig. 3.8.3   Rheumatoid nodules at the elbows.

- episcleritis
- fibrosing alveolitis
- Caplan's syndrome (rheumatoid lung nodules with associated pneumoconiosis)
- pericarditis
- vasculitis (vasculitic leg ulcers and mononeuritis multiplex)
- sensory neuropathy
- Felty's syndrome
  — RA
  — splenomegaly
  — pancytopenia
- amyloidosis (causes renal failure)
- anaemia (of chronic disorders).

Systemic lupus erythematosus

Much more common in women. Onset in early 20s.

Signs

- Arthritis
  — usually symmetrical, often migratory
  — affects the hands, wrists, elbows, knees and ankles
- Skin
  — photosensitivity
  — butterfly rash
  — Raynaud's phenomenon

— arteritic lesions
— alopecia
- Sjögren's syndrome
- Lung
  — alveolitis (crackles both sides)
  — pleural effusion
- Heart
  — pericarditis (rub)
  — myocarditis
  — Libman–Sachs endocarditis
- Kidneys
  — proteinuria
  — nephrotic syndrome
  — chronic renal failure
- Nervous system
  — cerebral lupus
    — confusion
    — intellectual impairment
    —psychiatric symptoms
  — mononeuritis multiplex
  — peripheral neuropathy.

Scleroderma

More common in females.

Signs

- Skin
  — tightened skin which is shiny, with loss of hair and pigmentation. (Try to pick up the skin on the back of the patient's hand between your thumb and index finger. This will be impossible.)
  — telangiectasia
  — facial appearance
    — tight skin
    — beaked nose
    — microstomia
  — Raynaud's phenomenon.
- Chest
  — alveolitis (basal crackles).

- Heart
  — pericarditis (rub)
  — congestive cardiac failure
  — conduction defects.
- Gut
  — oesophageal involvement (dysphagia)
  — small bowel involvement (malabsorption).
- Arthritis
  — small joints of the hand (usually).
- Renal
  — chronic renal failure ± hypertension.

Ankylosing spondylitis

Much more common in men. It usually presents in the 20s or 30s. Over 95% are HLA B27-positive.

Signs

- Fixed spine
  — thoracic kyphosis, loss of lumbar lordosis
  — hyperextension of neck (this results in the typical 'question mark' posture; see Fig. 3.8.4)
- Arthritis
  — large joint monoarthritis of the lower limb
  — sacroileitis (pelvis 'spring').

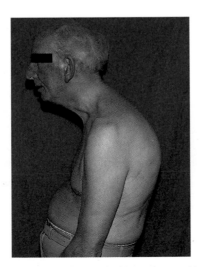

Fig. 3.8.4 The typical 'question mark' posture of ankylosing spondylitis.

X-ray

- Poor chest expansion
- Bamboo spine
- Sacroileitis.

Associations

- Aortic regurgitation
- Iritis, conjunctivitis
- Pulmonary fibrosis (apical)
- Mycetoma[†] (fungus ball in under-aerated upper lobe).

Sacroileitis may also be found in inflammatory bowel disease.

Psoriatic arthropathy

Affects men and women equally.

Signs

- Arthritis (there are three main patterns of joint involvement)
  — *terminal* interphalangeal joints (distinguishes it from RA), usually asymmetrical
  — *polyarthropathy* indistinguishable from RA, but seronegative
  — *arthritis mutilans*: resorption of phalangeal heads resulting in a destructive arthropathy of the hands
- Skin
  — psoriatic plaques
  — pitting of fingernails
  — onycholysis
  — scaling of scalp.

There are no rheumatoid nodules as this is a seronegative arthritis. The skin changes may be minimal, but patients will almost invariably have psoriatic nail changes. Remember that RA and psoriasis are common; not every patient with arthritis and psoriasis will have psoriatic arthropathy. These two conditions can coexist (see Figs 3.8.5 and 3.8.6).

Gout

Chronic gout

Chronic elevation of serum urate.

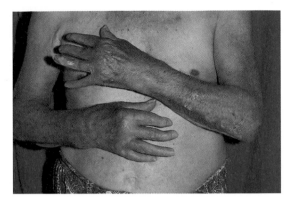

Fig. 3.8.5   Psoriatic arthropathy (arthritis mutilans). Note the patches of psoriasis at the elbows and deformity of the hands, including the distal interphalangeal joints.

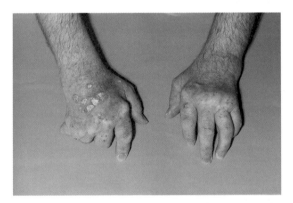

Fig. 3.8.6   Another combination of psoriatic skin lesions and a deforming arthritis of the hands. This time the arthritis is due to rheumatoid arthritis (distal interphalangeal joints relatively spared) and the psoriasis is an incidental finding.

Signs

- Gouty tophi
  — periarticular
  — pinna of ear
- Arthritis
  — osteoarthrosis (OA) of the affected joints.

Acute gout[†]

Signs

- Arthritis (asymmetrical)

- Great toe
- Wrist/elbow
- Any other joint may be affected.

Causes

- Idiopathic
- Thiazide diuretics
- Renal failure
- Psoriasis
- Myeloproliferative disorders.

Monoarthritis

Causes

- Trauma
- Sepsis
  — bacterial (including tuberculosis and gonorrhoea)
  — viral, e.g. rubella
- Seronegative arthritides
  — osteoarthrosis (OA)
  — psoriasis
  — ankylosing spondylitis (hip, knee)
  — Reiter's disease (ankle, knee)
  — gout
  — pseudogout (knee)
- RA (monoarthritis is an unusual but recognised mode of presentation)
- SLE, scleroderma
- Crohn's disease, ulcerative colitis (hip, knee, ankle).

Raynaud's phenomenon

Signs

- May be none (history important)
- Dystrophic changes ⎫
- Loss of the fingertips ⎬ Severe
- Nail changes ⎪ cases
- Frank digital gangrene. ⎭ only (see Fig. 3.8.7)

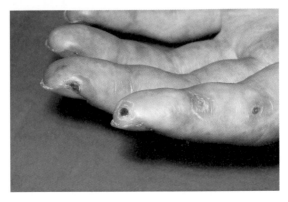

Fig. 3.8.7   Frank digital gangrene in a patient with severe Raynaud's disease.

Causes

- Raynaud's disease (idiopathic)
- Scleroderma
- RA, SLE
- Cervical rib
- Atherosclerotic
- Polycythaemia.

It is more common in people who use vibrating tools. Remember to look for scars in the root of the neck indicating that the patient has had a sympathectomy to alleviate the symptoms.

Marfan's

Arachnodactyly
Scoliosis
SUFE
Spondylolithesis
Flat feet
(A) valve dis
High palate
(A) aneurysm
Retinal detachment
Lens dislocation

Polymyositis

Muscles.
Arthritis
Raynaud's.
Dysphagia.
Sjogren's.

KEY QUESTIONS

RHEUMATOLOGY

1. **What are the causes of**
   - Raynaud's phenomenon
   - sacroileitis
   - gout
   - monoarthritis of the ankle?
2. **What are the differences radiologically between rheumatoid arthritis and osteoarthritis?**
3. **What are the systemic complications of rheumatoid arthritis?**
4. **What is Reiter's syndrome?**

3.9

Dermatology
N. J. Reynolds

Skin disease is very common but is not examined in detail in the Final MB exam. Candidates are presented with either common dermatological conditions or important dermatological manifestations of systemic disease. Remember, however, that dermatology may also be encountered in the viva, particularly with the use of clinical or histopathological photographs.

Medical students sometimes believe that dermatological diagnosis is reached through a 'picture matching' process and that the history is irrelevant. This is rarely the case. A logical approach to history and examination is essential. However, if presented with a dermatological long case I would recommend an initial brief examination of the skin, as the diagnosis may then be apparent, allowing a more appropriate and relevant history to be taken. In short cases, a logical examination, description of clinical findings, interpretation of physical signs and an appropriate differential diagnosis are much more likely to impress the examiner than the offer of a single diagnosis (which may be incorrect).

Scheme for history of skin conditions

Initial lesion(s)

- Site
- Duration
- Spread
- Exacerbating/relieving factors.

PMH

Associated conditions.

Drugs

Dermatological side-effects are very common, including from over-the-counter medicines. They may exacerbate pre-existing skin disease. Include previous topical therapy, as this may modify the clinical appearance.

SH

- Environmental factors — occupation and work environment, geographical factors including residence and travel abroad, sun exposure and relevant hobbies
- The impact of the skin condition on the patient's life must be assessed.

FH

Many skin conditions have an hereditary component.

Scheme for examination of the skin

Examine the whole skin surface including mouth, eyes and scalp in a long case. Ensure optimal lighting — bedside lighting is often inadequate. Look and then palpate. Assess:

- single or multiple lesions*
- colour
- surface change — ? scaling
- margin — ill or well defined
- temperature
- depth of lesion
- distribution.

Decide whether the pathological process is primarily epidermal (associated with surface change/scaling), dermal or involves the subcutis. For deeper lesions, assess whether they are fixed to underlying tissues and/or overlying skin.

Consider logically the differential diagnosis and if necessary apply broad categories: inherited, metabolic (rare with skin disease), inflammatory, infection, malignant disease (primary or secondary), drugs, etc.

The distribution of lesions may be extremely helpful in reaching a differential diagnosis. For example, consider external influences (including infection), if the condition appears asymmetrical. Remember, however, that naevoid lesions and blood vessel/ lymphatic processes may also result in asymmetrical lesions. Think about ultraviolet light if lesions are confined to exposed skin.

Descriptive terms

- Macule — flat lesion
- Papule — circumscribed raised lesion < 1 cm diameter
- Nodule — circumscribed raised lesion > 1 cm diameter
- Vesicle, bulla — fluid-filled lesion
- Pustule — pus-filled lesion.

TYPICAL CASES

DERMATOLOGY

- Psoriasis
- Dermatitis
- Lichen planus
- Bullous disorders
- Erythema nodosum
- Generalised hyperpigmentation
- Leg ulceration
- Malignant disease

Psoriasis

Very common. Look for:

- well defined scaly plaques (Fig. 3.9.1)
- guttate lesions
- evidence of the Köebner phenomenon (lesions induced by trauma; Fig. 3.9.1)
- nail changes (pitting and onycholysis)
- scalp involvement
- arthropathy.

Pustular psoriasis may be localised to hands and feet or generalised (Fig. 3.9.2). Ask about:

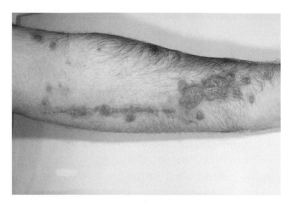

Fig. 3.9.1 Stable plaque psoriasis on forearm. Note linear lesion induced by local trauma (Köebner phenomenon).

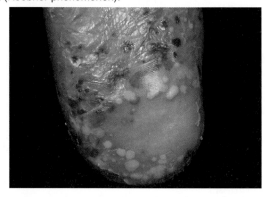

Fig. 3.9.2 Pustular psoriasis of feet. May also be generalised.

- exacerbating factors — sore throats (streptococcal infection)
- life events and stress
- skin trauma including sunburn
- FH
- previous therapy.

Dermatitis

May be due to atopic eczema, contact dermatitis, seborrhoeic dermatitis or varicose eczema (see below).

Atopic eczema

Very common. Onset often in early childhood but may persist into adulthood in more severe cases. Widespread, symmetrical ill-

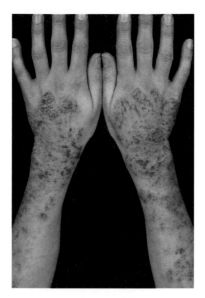

Fig. 3.9.3   Symmetrical ill-defined rash of atopic dermatitis persisting into adult life. Note that flexural involvement is not always seen.

defined areas of itchy red papulo-vesicles (Fig. 3.9.3), involving particularly the flexural aspects of elbows and knees. Xerosis and lichenification may be prominent.

Look for signs of topical steroid overusage, including epidermal atrophy, telangectasia and striae. Ask about:

* PH or FH of atopy
* exacerbating factors
* details of therapy.

Contact dermatitis

Uncommon. May be irritant or allergic in nature. Consider when 'eczema' is localised or asymmetrical (Fig. 3.9.4). Remember that allergic contact dermatitis can rarely occur on top of atopic eczema.

Ask about:

* occupation
* hobbies
* topical medicaments (Fig. 3.9.4).

Recommend patch testing if allergic contact dermatitis is suspected.

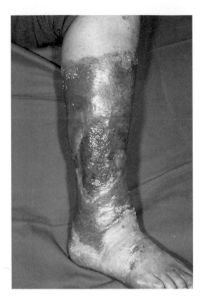

Fig. 3.9.4   Localised allergic contact dermatitis on right lower leg of a patient with venous ulceration. Note the sharp cut-off. Patch-testing demonstrated allergy to parabens, one of the components of medicated bandages.

Seborrhoeic dermatitis (Fig. 3.9.5)

Mild disease is common, but if severe consider HIV disease.

Varicose eczema

Always consider whether allergic contact dermatitis contributes to the clinical picture.

Lichen planus

Uncommon. Grouped, very itchy, violaceous flat-topped papules with white interlacing surface (Wickham's striae).
    Look for:

- nail changes — pterygium formation (Fig. 3.9.6)
- mucosal changes
- Köebner phenomenon.

Bullous disorders

Rare.

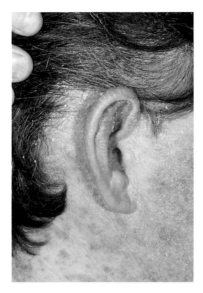

Fig. 3.9.5   Seborrhoeic dermatitis with scaling of the scalp and erythermatous scaly rash of face, chest and back.

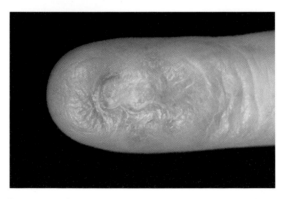

Fig. 3.9.6   Severe scarring and atrophy of nail in a patient with lichen planus. Note fusion of cuticle and nail bed (pterygium formation).

Pemphigoid

Subepidermal tense intact blisters on an inflammatory and often urticated base (Fig. 3.9.7). Age onset 65–75 years. Mucous membrane involvement is uncommon. Histology shows subepidermal bullae with an inflammatory infiltrate including eosinophils. Direct immunofluorescence shows deposition of immunoglobulin and C_3 along the basement membrane zone.

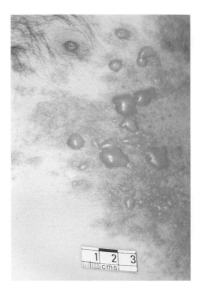

Fig. 3.9.7 Tense intact blisters on an erythematous base in bullous pemphigoid.

Pemphigus vulgaris

Intra-epidermal flaccid or deroofed blisters. Age onset 40–60 years. Mucous membrane involvement very common. Histology shows intra-epidermal bullae. Direct immunofluorescence shows deposition of immunoglobulin within the epidermis at keratinocyte junctions.

Dermatitis herpetiformis

Small, very itchy subepidermal blisters on extensor surfaces, particularly elbows, knees and buttocks — often excoriated (Fig. 3.9.8). Age of onset 20–55 years. Associated with gluten-sensitive enteropathy.

Other causes of bullous disorders

- Congenital (epidermolysis bullosa)
- Trauma
- Insect bite reaction
- Infections (staphylococcal scalded skin syndrome)
- Photosensitivity
- Drugs (barbiturates)
- Erythema multiforme.

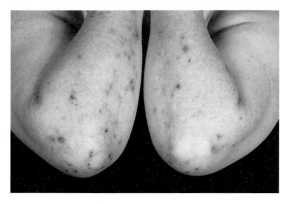

Fig. 3.9.8 Blisters are rarely seen in dermatitis herpetiformis. Note grouped excoriated papules over extensor aspect of elbow.

Erythema nodosum

Uncommon.

Causes

- Infections
  — streptococcal
  — TB
- Sarcoidosis
- Inflammatory bowel disease
- Drugs (sulphonamides).

Generalised hyperpigmentation

Uncommon.

Causes

- Addison's disease
- Malabsorption
- Haemochromatosis
- Drugs (chlorpromazine).

Leg ulceration

Very common.

Causes

- Venous (Fig. 3.9.4)
- Arterial
- Diabetic

- Vasculitis (rheumatoid arthritis)
- Malignant
- Pyoderma gangrenosum
- Sickle cell disease
- Necrobiosis lipoidica.

Ask about:

- intermittent claudication
- PH of DVT.

Assess:

- Edge of ulcer
- Distribution of ulcers (venous ulcers generally occur over medial and lateral malleoli)
- Arterial system — peripheral pulses
- Venous system — varicose veins
- Sensation — neuropathic ulcers
- Skin — varicose eczema.

Look for clues elsewhere (rheumatoid hands, for example). Necrobiosis lipoidica and pretibial myxoedema will be covered in chapter 3.10.

Malignant disease

May be primary or secondary.

Malignant melanoma (Fig. 3.9.9)

Uncommon but may come up in the viva. Distinguishing clinical features from a benign pigmented lesion are:

- history
  — changing size
  — changing colour
  — changing shape
  — itching
  — bleeding

- examination (Fig. 3.9.9)
  — diameter > 7 mm
  — irregular outline
  — asymmetry

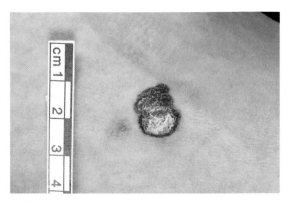

Fig. 3.9.9   Malignant melanoma. Note irregular margin, asymmetry, nodularity, surface change and irregular distribution of pigment.

— irregular distribution of pigment
— loss of normal surface markings
— oozing/crusting/bleeding/ulceration
— raised nodules.

Basal cell carcinoma

- Common
- Raised nodules with pearly edge and overlying telangectasia (Fig. 3.9.10)
- No precursor lesions
- Locally invasive but very rarely metastasize.

Squamous cell carcinoma

- Uncommon
- Raised keratinous lesions
- Precursor lesions include Bowens disease and actinic keratosis
- Metastases are not uncommon.

Cutaneous T-cell lymphoma (Mycosis fungoides)

- Rare
- Well defined *fixed* scaly plaques
- Look for associated poikiloderma (tclangectasia, epidermal atrophy and hyperpigmentation)
- May run an indolent course before progressing to tumour stage

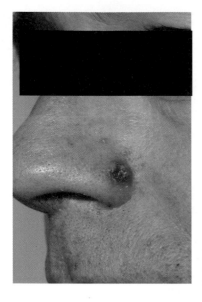

Fig. 3.9.10 Basal cell carcinoma in a characteristic site. Note raised pearly edge.

- Systemic involvement and lymphadenopathy is a late and often pre-terminal event
- May result in erythroderma with circulating atypical lymphocytes (Sézary cells) (very rare).

KEY QUESTIONS

DERMATOLOGY

1. With which condition is dermatitis herpetiformis associated?
2. What internal disorders may produce generalised pruritus?
3. How may contact dermatitis be distinguished from atopic dermatitis?
4. What are the cutaneous manifestations of internal malignancy?
5. How would you manage an erythrodermic patient?

3.10

Anatomical considerations: the upper limb, the lower limb, the face

You may be asked to examine part of the patient's anatomy, with no specific clues from the examiner as to which system contains the abnormal physical sign. This can wrong-foot the unwary candidate unless you specifically prepare yourself in advance. The three commonest areas asked about are:

1. the upper limb
2. the lower limb
3. the face.

The question may be: 'Examine this patient's hands' or 'Look at this patient's face'.

You will realise that, because of basic anatomical considerations, you will more than likely find the abnormality in the skin, nervous system or joints. Your examination should be tailored accordingly. Remember to inspect carefully. This may tell you where to concentrate your examination, or give you the diagnosis immediately. Don't forget to examine the peripheral pulses when examining the limbs.

QUESTIONS

The upper limb

If you are presented with an upper limb think of:
- skin
- joints
- nervous system.

The more common upper limb short cases are listed in Table 3.10.1. This is followed by some examples for you to consider. The answers are found towards the end of the chapter.

Table 3.10.1 Common upper limb short cases	
Skin (Chapter 3.9)	Psoriasis* Eczema* Lichen planus Dermatitis herpetiformis Scleroderma/Raynaud's
Joints (Chapter 3.8)	RA* OA* Psoriatic arthropathy SLE
Nervous system (Chapter 3.7)	Wasted hand* Ulnar nerve lesion Median nerve lesion Tremor
Miscellaneous	Clubbing* Palmar erythema Psoriatic nail changes Dupuytren's contracture Spider naevi

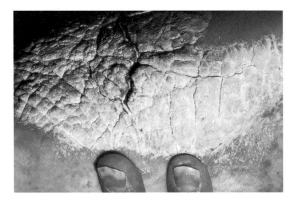

Fig. 3.10.1   (Answer on p. 157.)

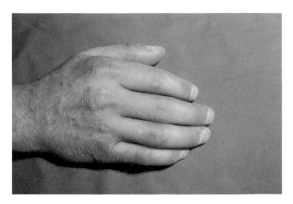

Fig. 3.10.2   (Answer on p. 157.)

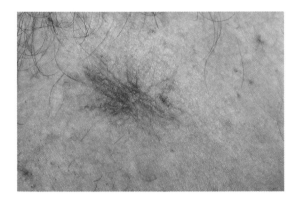

Fig. 3.10.3   (Answer on p. 157.)

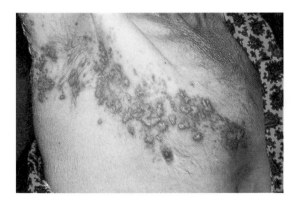

Fig. 3.10.4   (Answer on p. 158.)

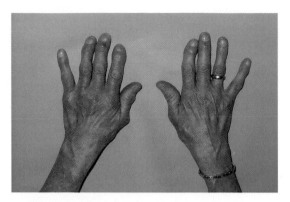

Fig. 3.10.5 (Answer on p. 158.)

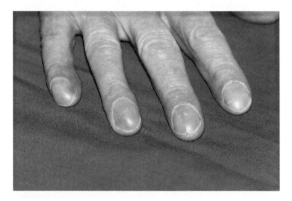

Fig. 3.10.6 (Answer on p. 158.)

The lower limb

Again, think of:
- skin
- joints
- nervous system.

Table 3.10.2 Common lower limb short cases

Skin	Leg ulcers*
	Psoriasis, dermatitis, etc.
	Pyoderma gangrenosum[†]
	Pre-tibial myxoedema[†]
	Necrobiosis lipoidica[†]
Joints	RA
	OA
	Charcot joint
Nervous system	Peripheral neuropathy*
	Spastic monoparesis*
	Spastic paraparesis
Miscellaneous	Bilateral pitting oedema*
	• CCF
	• hypoproteinaemia
	Unilateral swollen leg
	• cellulitis
	• DVT
	• ruptured Baker's cyst
	Peripheral arterial disease

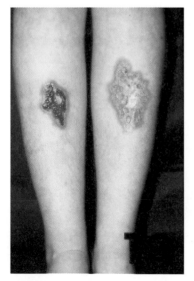

Fig. 3.10.7 (Answer on p. 158.)

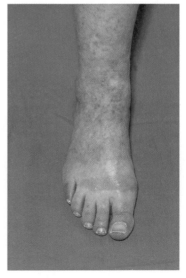

Fig. 3.10.8 (Answer on p. 158.)

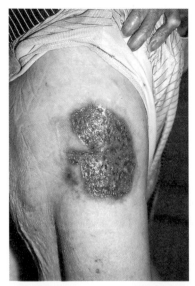

Fig. 3.10.9 (Answer on p. 158.)

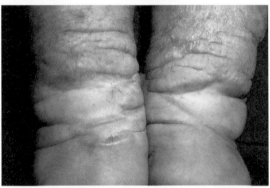

Fig. 3.10.10
(Answer on p. 158.)

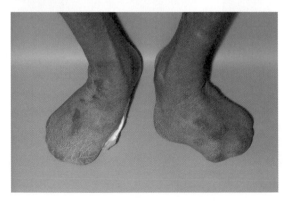

Fig. 3.10.11
(Answer on p. 158.)

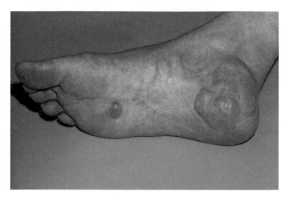

Fig. 3.10.12   (Answer on p. 159.)

The face

Rheumatological diseases are less common. Endocrinological disorders are more important.

Table 3.10.3 The face: common short cases		
Skin	Psoriasis, dermatitis, etc. Acne, rosacea	} Chapter 3.9
	SLE	Butterfly rash
	Scleroderma	Beaked nose, microstomia
	Herpes zoster	
	Alopecia	
	Xanthelasmata	Hyperlipidaemia
	Lupus pernio	Sarcoid nose
	Dermatomyositis	Heliotrope colour of eyelids
	Hereditary, haemorrhagic telangiectasia	Telangiectasia around mouth
Nervous system	Cranial nerve palsies Eye signs Parkinsonian facies	} Chapter 3.7
Endocrine system	Hypothyroidism Hyperthyroidism Acromegaly Cushing's syndrome	} See Chapter 3.6
Miscellaneous	Paget's disease	Frontal bossing
	Anaemia Jaundice	} See Chapter 3.4
	Saddle nose	Syphilis, Wegener's granulomatosis

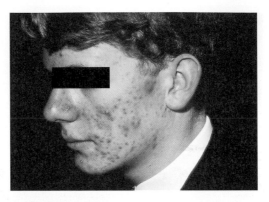

Fig. 3.10.13   (Answer on p. 159.)

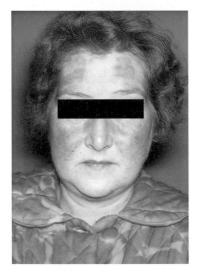

Fig. 3.10.14   (Answer on p. 159.)

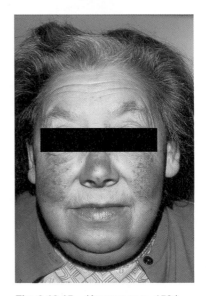

Fig. 3.10.15   (Answer on p. 159.)

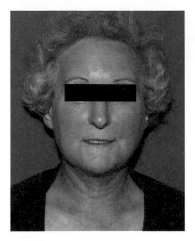

Fig. 3.10.16   (Answer on p. 159.)

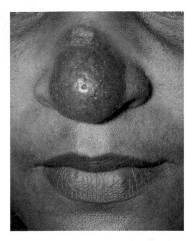

Fig. 3.10.17   (Answer on p. 159.)

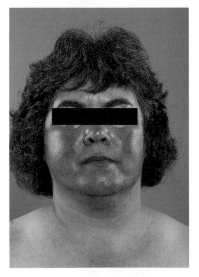

Fig. 3.10.18   (Answer on p. 159.)

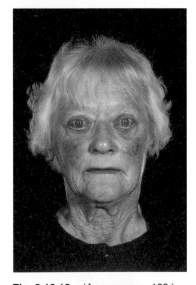

Fig. 3.10.19   (Answer on p. 159.)

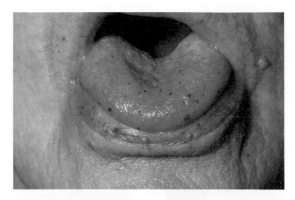

Fig. 3.10.20   (Answer on p. 160.)

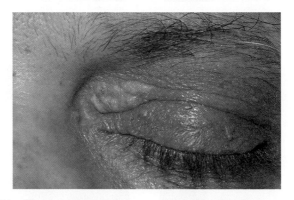

Fig. 3.10.21   (Answer on p. 160.)

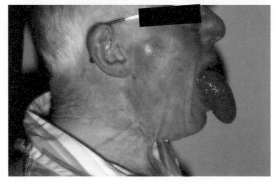

Fig. 3.10.22   (Answer on p. 160.)

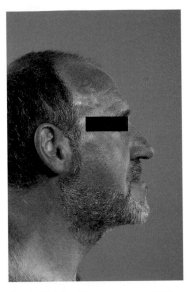

Fig. 3.10.23   (Answer on p. 160.)

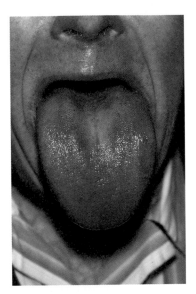

Fig. 3.10.24   (Answer on p. 160.)

ANSWERS

The upper limb

Figure 3.10.1

This is a case of plaque psoriasis. Note the onycholysis of the nails.

Figure 3.10.2

Scleroderma of hands. The skin on this patient's fingers is puffy, shiny and tethered down. There is some sclerodactyly (tapering of the fingers).

Figure 3.10.3

A spider naevus. These are always found in the area of the body drained by the superior vena cava (upper limb, head, neck and upper trunk). If you find more than three or four you should look carefully for other signs of chronic liver disease.

Figure 3.10.4

Herpes zoster affecting the T_2 dermatome.

Figure 3.10.5

Osteoarthrosis at the terminal interphalangeal joint. Note the Heberden's nodes and the deformity of the distal interphalangeal joint.

Figure 3.10.6

Clubbing of the fingernails.

The lower limb

Figure 3.10.7

Necrobiosis lipoidica. This is a rare complication of diabetes mellitus. Oval indurated plaques found on the shins. Note the brown/yellow margins and yellow waxy areas of atrophy.

Figure 3.10.8

Vitiligo. Very common. Associated with autoimmune conditions such as hypothyroidism, Addison's disease and diabetes mellitus (type 1).

Figure 3.10.9

Pyoderma gangrenosum. It is associated with RA and inflammatory bowel disease. It is found on the lower limb. Note the raised purplish margin and necrotic base.

Figure 3.10.10

Pre-tibial myxoedema. Very rare. Pink/skin coloured induration, areas of which have a 'peau d'orange' appearance. There is sometimes an associated hypertrichosis. Found in thyrotoxicosis.

Figure 3.10.11

This shows some of the complications of diabetes affecting the lower limb. There are bilateral toe amputations (peripheral arterial disease) and Charcot ankle joint (peripheral neuropathy). You can just make out the edge of a dressing on the right: this covers an infected, painless ulcer on the sole of the foot.

Figure 3.10.12

Neurofibromatosis (autosomal dominant). This patient's skin was covered with similar soft subcutaneous and pedunculated tumours. There is an increased incidence of meningioma, glioma and VIII nerve tumours. These benign tumours occasionally undergo sarcomatous change. Also look for café-au-lait patches (> 5), scoliosis and unilateral limb hypertrophy.

The face

Figure 3.10.13

Acne vulgaris.

Figure 3.10.14

Butterfly rash of systemic lupus erythematosus.

Figure 3.10.15

Myxoedema. Note the coarse features, 'peaches and cream' complexion and loss of outer third of the eyebrows.

Figure 3.10.16

Scleroderma. Note the tight skin, beaked nose and microstomia. This patient also demonstrates radial furrowing around the lips.

Figure 3.10.17

Lupus pernio. Sarcoidosis of the nose.

Figure 3.10.18

Cushing's syndrome.

Figure 3.10.19

Ophthalmopathy due to Graves' disease. This slide demonstrates true proptosis. (Reproduced by permission from Krentz A J 1997 Colour Guide: Diabetes. Churchill Livingstone, Edinburgh.)

Figure 3.10.20

Hereditary haemorrhagic telangiectasia. Autosomal dominant. These telangiectatic spots are found throughout the upper gastro-intestinal tract. The patient presents in middle age with iron deficiency anaemia and/or gastrointestinal haemorrhage.

Figure 3.10.21

Xanthelasma.

Figure 3.10.22

This patient has a huge tongue due to primary amyloidosis. Causes of a large tongue are:

- idiopathic
- carcinoma
- acromegaly
- amyloidosis.

Fig. 3.10.23

Acromegaly. This patient demonstrates proganthism and has a large nose. The supra-orbital ridges are not particularly pro-minent. Other features to look for include:

- large, burly stature
- spade-like hands and feet
- carpal tunnel syndrome
- organomegaly
- hypertension
- signs of cardiac failure
- bitemporal hemianopia
- large tongue.

Figure 3.10.24

As Figure 3.10.22.

3.11

The electrocardiogram (ECG)

You need to have a basic grasp of the ECG: you ought to be able to recognise simple abnormalities, e.g. myocardial infarction. Some medical schools specifically exclude ECG diagnosis from their clinical paper (I am not sure why). It is worthwhile finding out what emphasis is placed on ECGs in the exam you are sitting and tailoring your revision accordingly.

READING THE ECG

Look at each individual part of the ECG in turn, using the following list:

- rate
- rhythm
- axis
- P wave
- PR interval
- QRS complex
- ST segment
- T wave
- U wave
- pattern recognition.

Like most things in medicine it is best to start off with a routine and adhere rigidly to it, at least in the first instance. Look at as many ECGs as possible and read them using this scheme. You will eventually reach a point (perhaps in years to come) when a glance will be sufficient to tell you the diagnosis (by pattern recognition). Do not do this in the examination.

Note. On most ECGs with standard settings: one small square (1 mm) = 0.04 s; one large square (5 mm) = 0.2 s.

Rate

Simple. Measure the distance (in large squares) between two consecutive R waves and divide into 300, that is:

$$\frac{300}{\text{R–R interval}}$$

For example, if the R–R interval is four squares:

$$\text{Rate} = \frac{300}{4} = 75 \text{ beats/min}$$

Bradycardia: rate < 60; tachycardia: rate > 100.

Rhythm

This can be rather more tricky. Having said this I think it would be unfair for you to be shown a complex arrhythmia.

Normal sinus rhythm

There is a P wave before each QRS complex.
    PR interval < 0.2 s (five small squares).
    QRS complex width < 0.12 s (three small squares).

Ectopics (Fig. 3.11.1)

Ventricular. The QRS complex is wide (< 0.12 s) and bizarre in shape.
Atrial. The P wave is an unusual shape, or may be inverted. It will come slightly earlier or slightly later than expected. The QRS complex is normal width.

Tachyarrhythmias

Supraventricular. The width of the QRS complex is normal (i.e. < 0.12 s) and the rate > 100 beats/min.
(i) Sinus tachycardia. P wave before each QRS complex. R–R interval regular.
(ii) Supraventricular tachycardia. P waves may not be evident, e.g. nodal tachycardia, atrial tachycardia. Regular R–R interval.
(iii) Atrial fibrillation. No P waves. Irregularly irregular R–R interval. Irregular fibrillating pattern of baseline.

P WAVE ABNORMALITIES

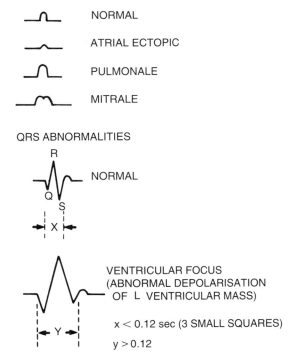

Fig. 3.11.1   P wave and QRS abnormalities.

Ventricular

(i) Ventricular tachycardia (VT).   Broad complex (QRS > 0.12 s). Tachyarrhythmia (rate > 100 beats/min). P wave impossible to see (usually).

Occasionally atrial beats can be conducted to the ventricles through an abnormal pathway at the a-v node. This can cause an SVT with aberrant conduction, which may be indistinguishable from VT. (This is postgraduate medicine.)

(ii) Ventricular fibrillation (VF).   Bizarre waveform with no discernible baseline or meaningful complexes. The patient will have no output ('cardiac arrest'). If the patient has a pulse then check the ECG leads, as one has probably fallen off.

Bradyarrhythmias

(i) Sinus bradycardia.   P waves are present and regular. Rate < 60 beats/min. Normal QRS configuration.

(ii) Nodal. No P waves at all. Rate < 60 beats/min. Normal QRS configuration.

(iii) Heart block (Fig. 3.11.2). This is caused by an increased refractory period of the a-v node (of varying degrees of severity). In complete heart block the a-v node will allow no electrical impulse to pass from the atria to the ventricles, which therefore function independently.

First degree (1°). PR interval > 0.2 s. All P waves followed by normal QRS.

Second degree (2°).

Wenckebach (Mobitz type I). PR interval gradually

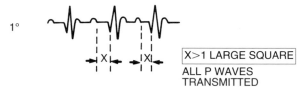

2° a) WENCKEBACH (MOBITZ TYPE I)

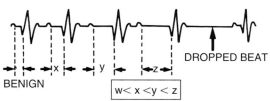

2° b) MOBITZ TYPE II

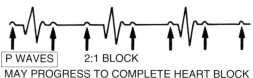

3° COMPLETE HEART BLOCK

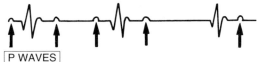

Fig. 3.11.2 Heart block.

increases in length until there is a dropped beat (atrial beat not transmitted to ventricles via a-v node).

Mobitz type II.   PR interval 0.2 s. Dropped beats (a-v conduction failure) are regular: e.g. two to one block (2:1) — alternate beats dropped; three to one block (3:1) — every third beat dropped. Mobitz type II has a more serious prognosis, as it often progresses to complete heart block.

Complete heart block (3°).   Complete a-v dissociation. P waves bear no relationship to QRS. QRS may be wide and bizarre-shaped. The rate may drop to a very low value (20 beats/min). This causes reduced cardiac output and syncope.

Axis

Easy, if you know how. Use the diagram of electrical vectors (Fig. 3.11.3) and the standard leads (I, II, III, AVF, AVL, AVR) of Case 1 (see 'typical cases' later in chapter).

Find the *isoelectric lead* (i.e. the one in which the size of the R wave is most equivalent to the size of the S wave). In Case 1 it is lead AVF. Check this against the diagram of electrical vectors (Fig. 3.11.3). In this instance the isoelectric vector will be at approximately +90°. Now look at the ECG again and find the lead(s) with the greatest positive deflection (i.e. the largest R waves). In Case 1, this is I and AVL.

The electrical axis of the heart will be at 90° to the isoelectric lead in the direction of the large R waves: electrical axis (Case 1) = 0°; normal axis ranges from +90° to –30°.

P wave (Fig. 3.11.1)

It should be less than 2.5 mm tall. It is tallest in lead II and it is for this reason that lead II is often used as the rhythm strip:

- 'P' mitrale (mitral valve disease) — double-topped P wave due to left atrial enlargement
- 'P' pulmonale (pulmonary hypertension) — large single-peaked P wave due to right atrial enlargement.

PR interval

From the start of the P wave to the start of the R wave should be 0.12–0.2 s (three to five small squares).

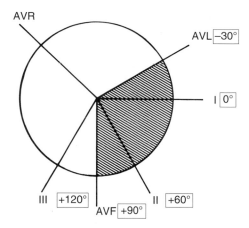

Fig. 3.11.3 Electrical axis. The shaded area represents the normal range of electrical axis.

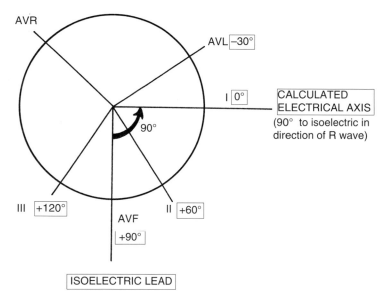

Fig. 3.11.4 Working out the electrical axis. The calculation of electrical axis in this diagram refers to the ECG of Case 1, to be found later in this chapter.

- PR > 0.2 s = first-degree heart blocks
- PR < 0.12 s is seen in the re-entrant tachycardias, e.g. Wolff–Parkinson–White syndrome.

QRS complex

Q waves

Q waves are normally seen in AVR. They are sometimes seen in III in normal individuals. Pathological Q waves are greater than 1 mm × 1 mm and denote transmural infarction of the myocardium.

R waves

The R wave should get bigger as you go across the V leads, V1–6. There is often little or no R wave in V1.

Causes of large R wave in V1 are:

- dextrocardia
- pulmonary embolus
- right ventricular hypertrophy
- Wolff–Parkinson–White (type A)
- true posterior myocardial infarction.

In Wolff–Parkinson–White syndrome (W–P–W) the R wave has a slurred upstroke (delta wave) due to abnormal conduction of impulses through the a-v node via an aberrant pathway (see Fig. 3.11.5). These patients are prone to tachyarrhythmias such as atrial fibrillation.

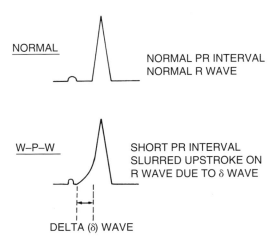

Fig. 3.11.5 The delta wave.

S wave

The S wave should get smaller as you traverse the V leads (V1–V6).

Bundle branch block (BBB)

Here the QRS complex is wide (> 0.12 s). In right BBB the QRS complex will be mainly upright in V1 and V2. In left BBB the QRS complex will be mainly upright in leads V5 and 6. LBBB makes the rest of the ECG uninterpretable (see 'typical cases').

ST segment

This should be normally at the same level as the baseline.

Raised ST segment

- Convex upwards
  — acute myocardial infarction
  — some normal negroes
- Concave upwards
  — pericarditis (especially in leads V5, 6, I and AVL).

Depressed ST segment

- Acute myocardial ischaemia
- Digoxin effect (see Fig. 3.11.6).

Note. The 'digoxin effect' does not imply digoxin toxicity, but simply that the patient is currently taking digoxin.

T wave

Peaked T wave

- Myocardial ischaemia
- Hyperkalaemia.

Peaked T waves are occasionally seen in the very early stages of acute myocardial infarction.

Inverted T wave

- Myocardial ischaemia
- Post-myocardial infarction

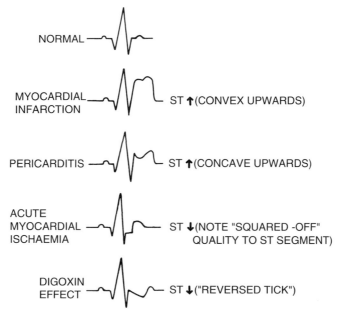

Fig. 3.11.6   Abnormal ST segments.

- Hypokalaemia
- Left ventricular hypertrophy/strain
- Following bundle branch block pattern.

U waves

Seen after the T wave as a little blip on the baseline.

Causes

- Normal fit young adults
- Myocardial ischaemia
- Hypokalaemia.

Pattern recognition

Essentially this means synthesising all the information you have gleaned from going through the above scheme. You should try to fit all the abnormalities together to make a diagnosis.

Experts can glance at an ECG and make an immediate diagnosis. This comes from years of practice perfecting their pattern recognition skills. You may find such people rather irritating — don't worry, you will be able to do it in the end, it's just a matter of enough practice.

TYPICAL CASES

This section gives you a chance to read specimen ECGs, similar to the ones you may be presented with during the examination. I suggest that you read them in the way I have demonstrated. The answers are to be found on the following page.

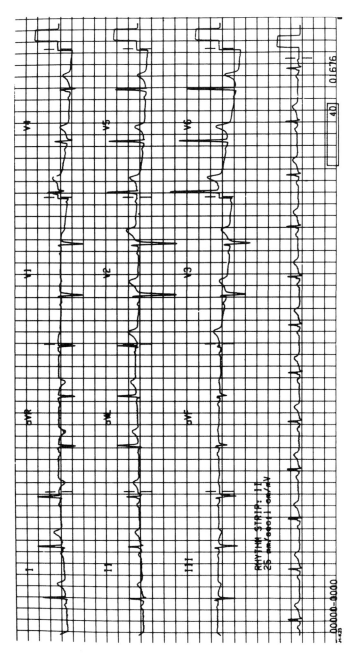

Case 1

Case 1

Rate:	75/min
Rhythm:	Sinus rhythm
Axis:	0°
P wave:	Normal
PR interval:	0.12 s
QRS complex:	Normal
ST segment:	Normal
T waves:	Normal
	(Note inverted T waves in V1, AVR and III. This is normal.)
U waves:	Absent
Pattern recognition:	Normal ECG

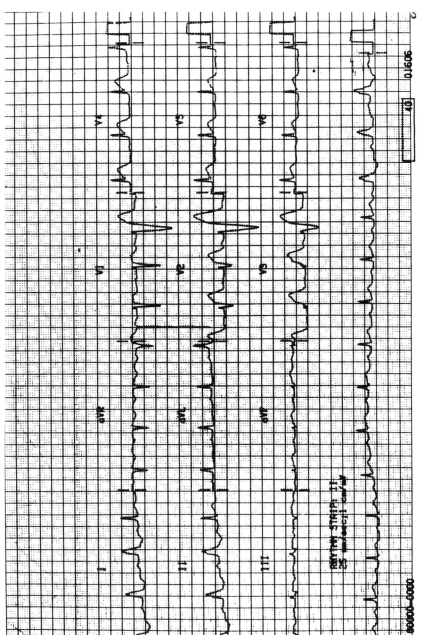

Case 2

Case 2

Rate:	80/min
Rhythm:	Sinus
Axis:	0°
P wave:	Normal
PR interval:	0.2 s (upper limit of normal)
QRS complex:	One ventricular ectopic (V1–3) Broad-looking complexes I, II
ST segment:	Raised V2–6
T wave:	Prominent V2–5
U wave:	Absent
Pattern recognition:	Acute anterior myocardial infarction

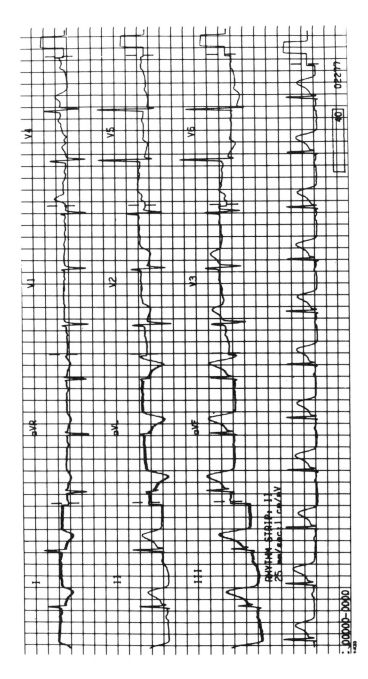

Case 3

Case 3

Rate:	70/min
Rhythm:	Sinus
Axis:	+60°
P wave:	Normal
PR interval:	0.16 s
QRS complex:	Normal
ST segment:	Raised ST II, III, AVF Depressed ST V5, 6, I, AVL
T wave:	Inverted V4–6, I, AVL
U wave:	Present V4–6
Pattern recognition:	Acute inferior myocardial infarction, with associated anterolateral myocardial ischaemia

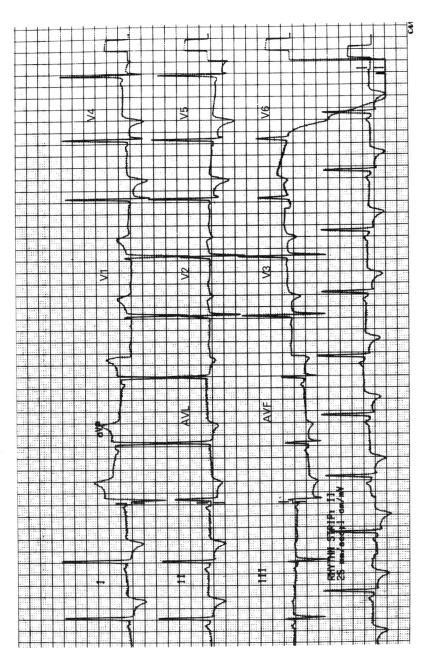

Case 4

Case 4

Rate:	60/min
Rhythm:	Sinus
Axis:	+15°
P wave:	Normal
PR interval:	0.12 s
QRS complex:	Large R waves V2–6, I, II Deep S waves V1–3 R wave V5 + S wave V1 = 49 mm
ST segment:	Widespread depression
T wave:	Inverted V2–6, I, II, AVL, AVF
U wave:	Absent
Pattern recognition:	Left ventricular hypertrophy

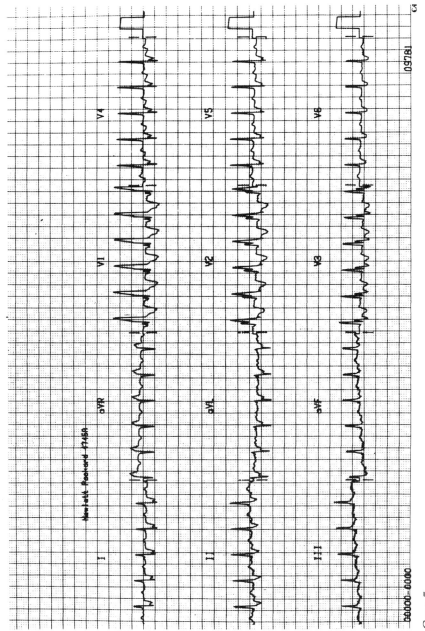

Case 5

Case 5

Rate:	150/min
Rhythm:	Atrial fibrillation
Axis:	+90°
P wave:	Absent
QRS complex:	Wide complexes V1–3 'M' pattern
ST segment:	Depressed V1–3
T wave:	Inverted V1–3
U wave:	Absent
Pattern recognition:	1. RBBB 2. Sinus tachycardia, cause unknown

Note. ST segment and T wave changes are secondary to RBBB.

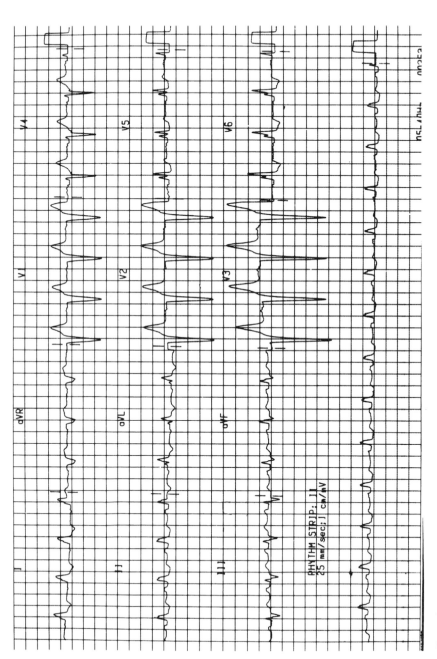

RHYTHM STRIP: II
25 mm/sec; 1 cm/mV

Case 6

Case 6

Rate:	85/min
Rhythm:	Sinus
Axis:	+30°
P wave:	Rather broader than normal
PR interval:	0.16 s
QRS:	Wide Bizarre-looking 'M' pattern V5–6
ST segment:	Depressed I, II, AVF, AVL, V5–6
T waves:	Inverted V5, V6, I, II, AVL
U waves:	Absent
Pattern recognition:	LBBB, aetiology unknown

Note. The ST segment and T wave abnormalities are secondary to LBBB.

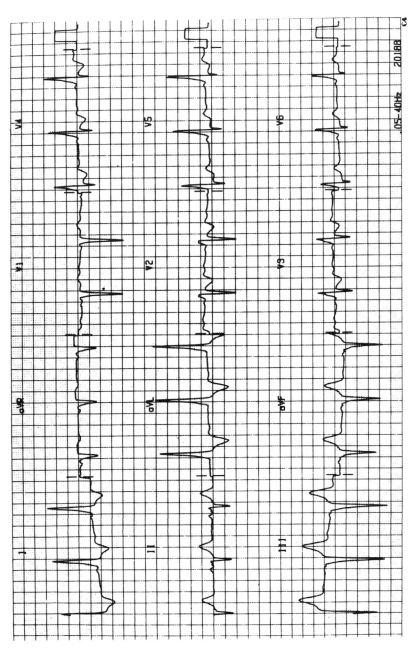

Case 7

Case 7

Rate:	65/min
Rhythm:	Sinus
Axis:	−60° (left axis deviation)
P wave:	Normal
PR interval:	0.1 s (abnormally short)
QRS complex:	Abnormal-looking Width 0.12 s Slurred upstroke to R wave (delta wave)
ST segment:	Depressed V2–6, I, AVL
T wave:	Inverted V2–4, I, AVL
U waves:	Absent
Pattern recognition:	Wolff–Parkinson–White syndrome

Note. This ECG bears a striking similarity to LBBB (Case 6).

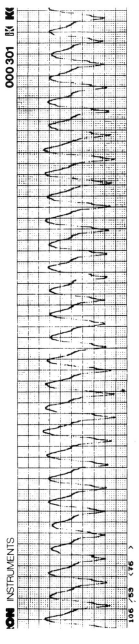

Case 8

Case 8

Broad complex tachycardia.

Rate: 150/min

Diagnosis: Ventricular tachycardia (VT)

This may be impossible to distinguish from SVT with aberrant conduction without doing sophisticated electrophysiological studies (see main text).

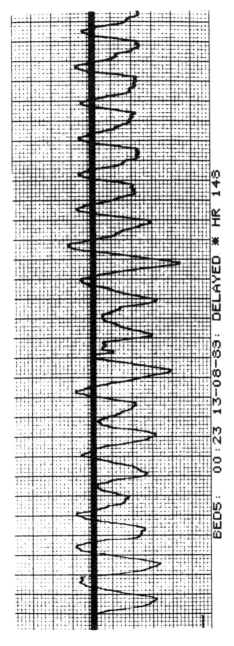

BED5:   00:23 13-08-83: DELAYED * HR 148

Case 9

Case 9

Broad complex trace with no discernible underlying rhythm.

Patient pulseless.

Diagnosis: Ventricular fibrillation (VF)

Call the cardiac arrest team.

ECG

I have made it easy this time by including the answers.

1. **ECG changes in pulmonary embolus★:**
   - none★
   - sinus tachycardia
   - RBBB
   - S1, Q3, T3[†] (S wave in I, Q wave in III, inverted T in III).
2. **ECG changes in myocardial infarction★:**
   - none
   - hyperacute, peaked T waves
   - ST elevation
   - Q waves
   - T wave inversion.

   These changes occur over the first 36 hours. Q waves and T wave inversion may persist.
3. **Arrhythmias in myocardial infarction★.**
   The answer to this is easy: any (see earlier in this chapter).
4. **Causes of sinus bradycardia★:**
   - vasovagal syncope
   - fit young athletes
   - post-myocardial infarction
   - iatrogenic (β blocker)
   - raised intracranial pressure ⎫
   - myxoedema   ⎬ rare
   - jaundice   ⎪
   - hypothermia.   ⎭
5. **Causes of sinus tachycardia★:**
   - anxiety
   - pain
   - post-myocardial infarction
   - iatrogenic (β agonists)
   - pulmonary embolus
   - shock (of any aetiology)
   - thyrotoxicosis
   - fever.

6. **ECG effects of digoxin*:**
   - 'reversed tick' sign (Fig. 3.11.6)
   - a-v block
   - any arrhythmia, but especially electrical bigeminy and paroxysmal atrial tachycardia, with block (digoxin toxicity).

7. **Hypokalaemia*:**
   - prominent U wave
   - inverted T wave
   - ST depression
   - PR prolongation (see Fig. 3.11.7).

8. **Hyperkalaemia*:**
   - tall, peaked T wave
   - QRS widening
   - absent P wave (see Fig. 3.11.7).

9. **The ECG differences between pericarditis and pericardial effusion:**
   - pericarditis — ST elevation (concave upwards) V4–5, I, AVL (Fig. 3.11.6)
   - pericardial effusion — small-voltage ECG (all leads).

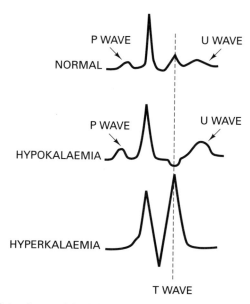

Fig. 3.11.7 Potassium and the ECG.

10. The ECG criteria for left ventricular hypertrophy (LVH):

- tall R waves V5, 6
- deep S waves V1, 2

(*Note*. If the height of the R wave in V6 plus the depth of the S wave in V1 is greater than 40 mm, this is definite evidence of LVH.)

- inverted T waves (sometimes) V4–6
- LAD.

11. Causes of left axis deviation (LAD) (axis –30° to –120°):

- left anterior hemiblock
- inferior myocardial infarction
- chronic obstructive airways disease
- Wolff–Parkinson–White syndrome
- left ventricular hypertrophy.

12. Cause of right axis deviation (RAD) (axis +90° to +180°):

- right ventricular hypertrophy
- dextrocardia
- Wolff–Parkinson–White syndrome
- left posterior hemiblock (diagnosed by excluding the others)
- leads on wrong way round.

13. Causes of LBBB (always an abnormal finding):

- ischaemic heart disease
- hypertension
- aortic valve disease
- following cardiac surgery.

14. Causes of RBBB:

- pulmonary embolism
- ischaemic heart disease
- atrial septal defect
- chronic pulmonary hypertension
- myocarditis
- some normal patients.

3.12

Radiology

The radiographs you may be asked to comment on during the course of the clinical examination or viva will not be complicated or too exotic — this would be unfair.

You need to try to demonstrate several things to the examiner. Firstly, appear as though you are familiar with looking at radiographs. Secondly, show that you have a logical, methodical approach to their interpretation. Finally, demonstrate that you can spot gross abnormalities, even if you are unsure what they represent.

To achieve these aims you need to practise looking at some radiographs, of the kind which crop up in the examination, using a systematic approach to their interpretation.

Approach to the chest radiograph

1. Always view on a well-lit viewing box

2. Look at the side marker (L or R)

This is to make sure that the radiograph has been put up the correct way round. There are several causes of an 'R' marker on the left of a chest radiograph:

- radiograph put on the viewing box the wrong way round
- radiograph marked incorrectly by the radiographer
- dextrocardia.

In the latter two cases the 'R' marker is on the same side as the cardiac apex.

3. Check name and date of birth

They may give important clues.

4. Determine whether the radiograph is a postero-anterior (PA) or anteroposterior (AP)

In PA views the cardiothoracic ratio (ratio of the transverse size of the cardiac outline to the transverse size of the thoracic cage) is normally less than 0.5. An AP projection will cause an apparent increase in this ratio (where none actually exists) because of the way in which the radiograph has been taken. Therefore, you must *never* comment on the cardiothoracic ratio of an AP chest radiograph.

If an AP view has been taken the radiographer should label the film 'AP' (see Case 9). This can be checked by looking at the position of the scapulae on the film. In an AP projection the scapulae overlie the lung fields, but in a good-quality PA view they should not (compare Cases 9 and 10).

5. View the radiograph as a whole

Your eye may be caught by a gross abnormality.

6. View each part of the radiograph in turn

Ignore the temptation to blurt out your first impression. You must now methodically look at each part of the radiograph in turn, to see if you can spot any other abnormalities. I use the following scheme:

- soft tissues
  - breasts
  - subcutaneous tissues
    - chest
    - neck
    - arms
- bony structures
  - humeri
  - scapulae
  - clavicles
  - cervical/thoracic spine
  - ribs
- pleura and diaphragm
- mediastinal structures
- lung fields.

7. Take another look at the radiograph as a whole

8. Synthesise

Now synthesise the above steps, to arrive at your answer. Remember to relate the radiological findings to any clinical information you already know about the patient. Try to illustrate to the examiner that you have looked at the radiograph methodically. For example:

Question:	'What abnormalities do you see on this chest radiograph?'
Bad answer (although correct):	'Carcinoma of the bronchus.'
Good answer:	'There is a 4 cm nodule in the mid-zone of the left lung field. This has a slightly irregular margin. The superior edge is particularly indistinct, with linear shadows radiating into the left upper lobe. The most likely cause for this appearance would be carcinoma of the bronchus. I can see no evidence of metastatic spread to the bones, mediastinal structures or other lung field, which all appear normal.'

This general approach can be applied to any radiograph, including contrast radiology. Once you have got the general idea, all you need is practice.

SPECIMEN CASES

I have included some radiological cases for you to consider. The answers are to be found towards the end of the chapter.

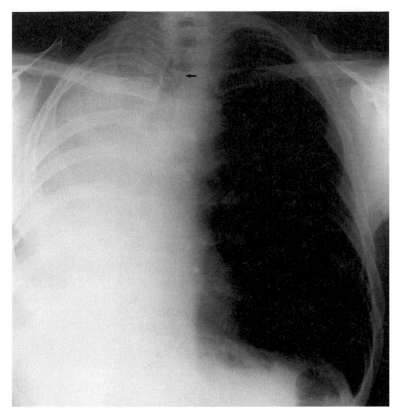

Case 1 (answer on p. 216)

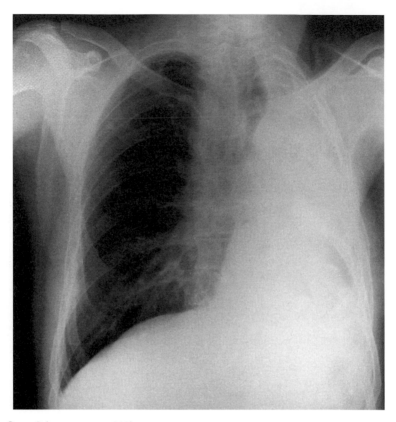

Case 2 (answer on p. 216)

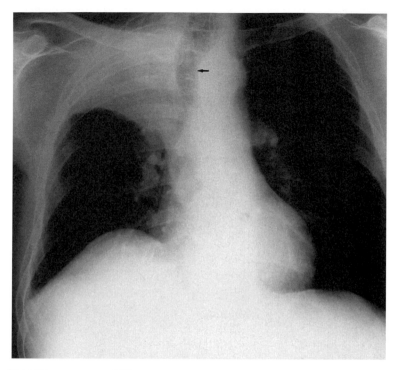

Case 3 (answer on p. 217)

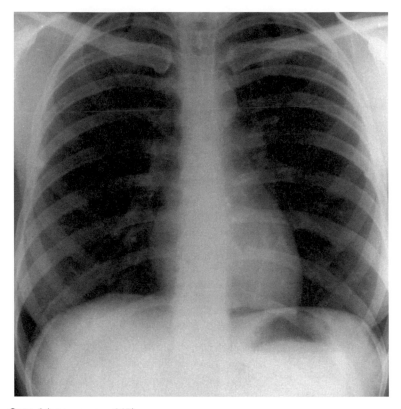

Case 4 (answer on p. 217)

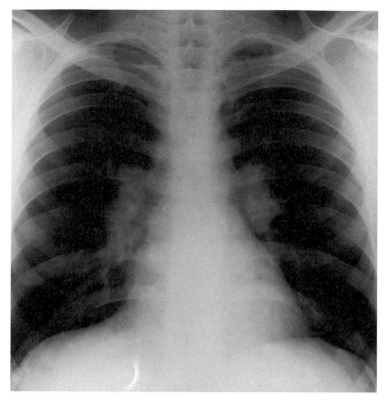

Case 5 (answer on p. 217)

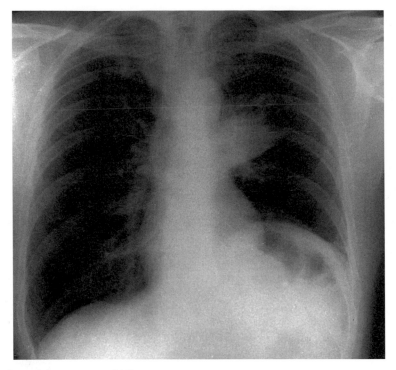

Case 6 (answer on p. 218)

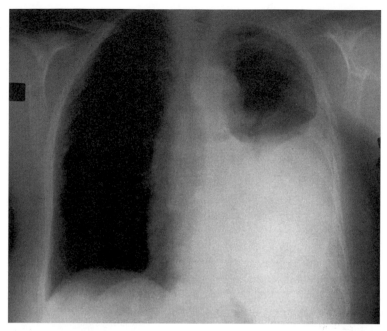

Case 7 (answer on p. 218)

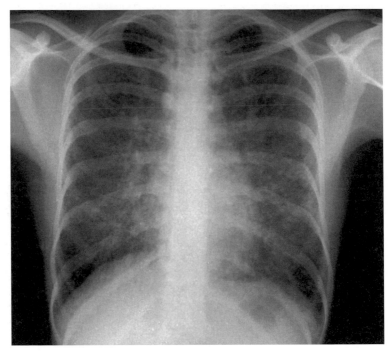

Case 8 (answer on p. 219)

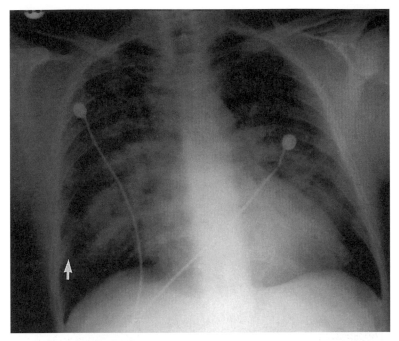

Case 9 (answer on p. 219)

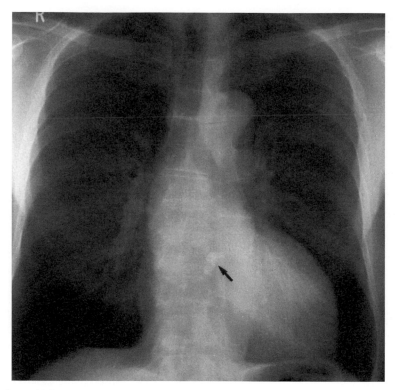

Case 10 (answer on p. 220)

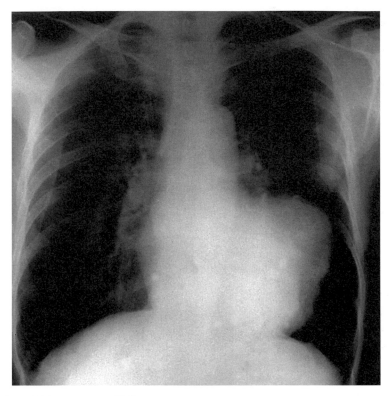

Case 11 (answer on p. 220)

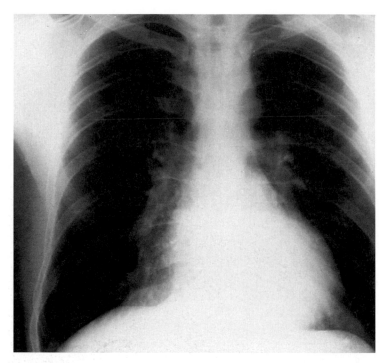

Case 12 (answer on p. 221)

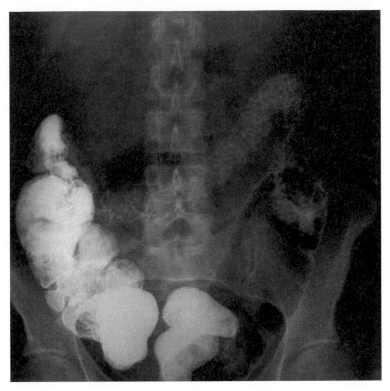

Case 13 (answer on p. 221)

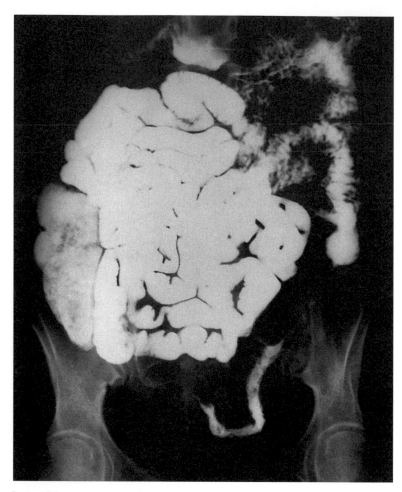

Case 14 (answer on p. 222)

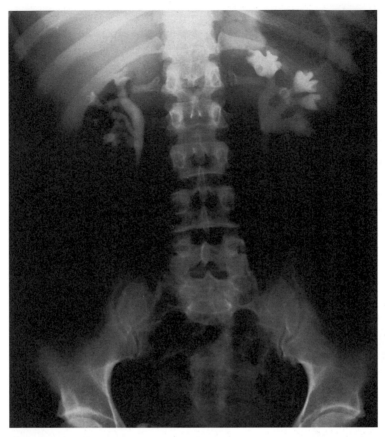

Case 15a (answer on p. 222)

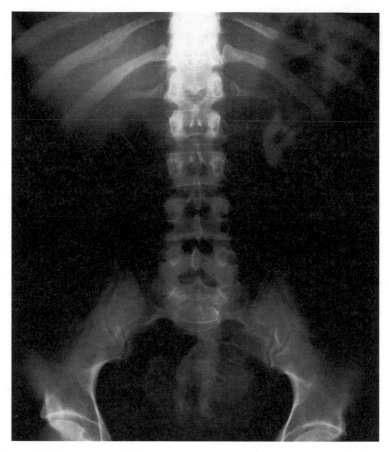

Case 15b (answer on p. 223)

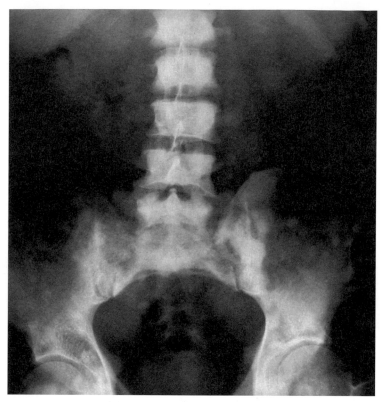

Case 16 (answer on p. 223)

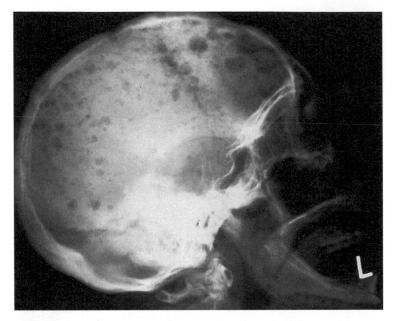

Case 17 (answer on p. 224)

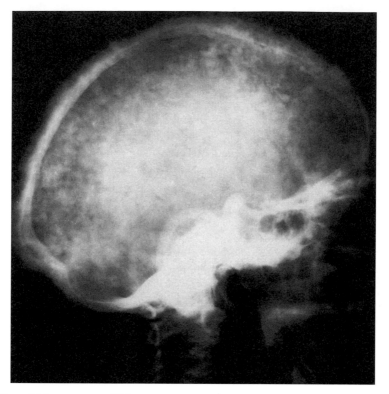

Case 18 (answer on p. 224)

ANSWERS TO SPECIMEN CASES

Case 1

This is a PA chest radiograph.
The whole of the right lung field is radio-opaque ('white-out').
The arrow indicates the left margin of the trachea. This, together with the position of the cardiac outline (which is barely visible), implies mediastinal shift to the right, due to loss of lung volume on this side.
The right fifth rib is absent.
Soft tissues — normal.
Conclusion. Post-pneumonectomy chest radiograph.

Case 2

This is a PA chest radiograph.
The whole of the left lung field is radio-opaque.
There is considerable loss of volume of the left lung (tracheal and mediastinal deviation to the left).
Bony structures — normal.
Soft tissues — normal.
Conclusion. Collapse, left lung. In this case it was due to a large carcinoma of the bronchus obstructing the left main bronchus. This was confirmed at bronchoscopy.

Case 3

This is a PA chest radiograph.
The right lung has a homogeneous radio-opaque area in the upper zone. This has a sharply demarcated lower edge, convex upwards, which is almost certainly an abnormally high horizontal fissure.
The trachea is pulled over to the right.
The right hemidiaphragm is domed medially, and slightly higher than normal.
Bony structures — normal.
Soft tissues — normal.
Conclusion.   Partial collapse, right upper lobe.

Case 4

This is a normal PA chest radiograph.

Case 5

This is a PA chest radiograph.
There is bilateral hilar lymphadenopathy.
In addition to this there is also paratracheal lymphadenopathy (look adjacent to the trachea, just below the medial end of the right clavicle).
Lung fields — normal.
Pleura — normal.
Bones — normal.
Soft tissues — normal.
Conclusion.   Bilateral hilar lymphadenopathy. Possible causes:

- sarcoidosis
- tuberculosis
- lymphoma.

Case 6

This is a PA chest radiograph.
There is a mass at the hilum. Its inferior surface is well demarcated, but its superior and lateral edges are irregular. Its medial surface merges with the mediastinal structures.
There is a raised left hemidiaphragm.
Right lung — normal.
Bony structures — normal.
Soft tissues — normal.
Conclusion. Carcinoma of the bronchus causing a left phrenic nerve palsy.

The phrenic nerve palsy can be confirmed radiologically by fluoroscopic screening of the diaphragm.

Case 7

This is a PA chest radiograph.
There is homogeneous shadowing in the lower and mid-zones of the left lung field. The superior border is well demarcated and concave upwards.
The left costophrenic angle has been obscured.
The mediastinum is central.
The right lung field is normal.
The left breast is absent.
Bony structures — normal.
Conclusion. Left pleural effusion.

Subsequent investigation revealed it to be due to metastatic adenocarcinoma. The primary was removed from the left breast 8 years previously.

Case 8

This is a PA chest radiograph.
There are small nodules (1–2 cm diameter) and fine line
shadows spread evenly throughout both lung fields
(reticulonodular shadowing). There is, possibly, relative
sparing of the apices.
Mediastinal structures — normal.
Pleura/diaphragm — normal.
Bony structures — normal.
Soft tissues — normal.
Conclusion.   Reticulonodular shadowing, cause unknown.

There are many possible causes, including:

* miliary tuberculosis
* sarcoidosis
* pneumoconiosis
* lymphangitis carcinomatosa.

Case 8 was due to sarcoidosis.

Case 9

This is an AP chest radiograph. Note the position of the
medial border of the scapulae, which commonly project over
the edge of the lung fields in an AP film.
There is fluffy shadowing in both lung fields, particularly in
the mid-zones. The upper lobe vessels are bulky. There are
Kerley B lines (arrowed at the right base). ECG leads are
present.
Soft tissues — normal.
Pleura and diaphragm — normal.
Bony structures — normal.
Conclusion.   Pulmonary oedema.

NB.   You cannot comment on the cardiac size on this film,
even though it looks large, as it is an AP view.

Case 10

This is a PA chest radiograph.
The cardiothoracic ratio is 0.52, which is just above the normal limit. There is an area of calcification overlying the cardiac silhouette (arrowed). This represents a calcified aortic valve, although it is impossible to say this with certainty without doing a lateral view.
The lung fields contain a generalised increase in vascular markings, and in particular the upper lobe blood vessels look bulky.
Soft tissues — normal.
Pleura and diaphragm — normal.
Bony structures — normal.
Conclusion.   Calcific aortic stenosis, with secondary increase in pulmonary venous pressure.

Case 11

This is a PA chest radiograph.
Cardiothoracic ratio = 0.56 (abnormal).
There is cardiomegaly. The main area of cardiac enlargement is on the left side of the cardiac outline, which also appears to have a double shadow. The left border of the heart is considerably 'bowed-out' (convex outwards).
Lung fields — normal.
Soft tissues — normal.
Pleura and diaphragm — normal.
Bony structures — normal.
Conclusion.   Left ventricular enlargement due to a cardiac aneurysm.

Case 12

This is a PA chest radiograph.
Mediastinum — normal.
Lung fields — normal.
Soft tissues — normal.
Pleura and diaphragm — normal.
Bony structures — abnormal.
Conclusion. This radiograph demonstrates classical rib notching, as found in coarctation of the aorta. This is seen on the inferior surfaces of the ribs, overlying the mid-zones of both lung fields.

This radiograph does not demonstrate the other radiological feature of coarctation — post-stenotic dilatation of the aorta. This would be seen as an enlargement of the mediastinal shadow in the area between the aortic knuckle and the left hilum. This case illustrates the necessity of looking carefully and methodically at all areas of the radiograph.

Case 13

This is a barium enema examination.
The transverse colon shows a grossly abnormal appearance. Throughout the whole of the transverse and proximal descending colon there is severe and continuous mucosal ulceration and oedema. There is loss of the normal haustral pattern in this region. The abnormalities show relative sparing of the ascending colon.
Conclusion. These findings are in keeping with the diagnosis of ulcerative colitis.

Case 14

This is a small bowel contrast study.

Barium outlines the small bowel. In addition there is a small amount of contrast in the stomach and duodenal cap (top of the picture).

There is an area of stricturing of the small bowel (overlying the left sacroiliac joint). Proximal to this there is a short length of bowel with abnormal mucosa. This demonstrates mucosal oedema and ulceration, including several 'rose-thorn' ulcers.

Conclusion.   These findings are compatible with Crohn's disease.

Case 15a

This is an intravenous urogram (IVU).

Contrast is seen in both pelvicalyceal systems and proximal ureters.

The left ureter can just be seen in the pelvis.

The left pelvicalyceal system is slightly dilated, compared with the right.

Bladder — not seen.

Bony structures — normal.

Soft tissues — normal.

Conclusion.   Slight enlargement of the left pelvicalyceal system, cause unknown.

If you are asked to comment on an IVU always ask to see a control film (a plain radiograph, before contrast was given). Please see Case 15b.

Case 15b

This is a control film for the IVU shown in Case 15a, and was therefore taken before the injection of contrast. The cause of the minimal dilatation of the left pelvicalyceal system is now obvious. There is a large staghorn calculus on the left.

Note.   It is impossible to make this diagnosis from the IVU alone, without seeing the control film.

Case 16

This is a plain radiograph of the pelvis.
There are sclerotic deposits throughout the lumbar spine and pelvis.
Conclusion.   This appearance is seen in carcinoma of:

- prostate
- breast
- thyroid.

Case 17

This is a lateral skull radiograph.
There are multiple circular defects of varying sizes throughout the vault of the skull. These also affect the mandible.
Conclusion. This is a characteristic appearance of multiple myeloma.

NB. Causes of 'holes' in the vault of the skull include:

- congenital
- malignant tumours
  — myeloma
  — metastatic carcinoma
  — lymphoma
- benign tumours
  — neurofibroma
- arteriovenous malformations.

Case 18

This is a lateral skull radiograph.
There are multiple, fluffy opacities throughout the skull.
Conclusion. This 'cotton wool' effect is characteristic of Paget's disease.

PART 4

THE VIVA VOCE

The viva voce
Key questions

4

The viva voce

THE VIVA VOCE

The primary purpose of this exercise is to test a student's problem-solving ability. Most general physicians will also use this opportunity to check that the student is familiar with the management of medical emergencies. Questions are therefore frequently asked by the examiner describing a clinical scenario, followed by direct questions which often relate to medical management issues.

An example of this type of question would be as follows:

'You are called to the Accident and Emergency department to see a 25-year-old woman. She appears to be deeply unconscious. How would you manage this patient?'

This type of question can appear daunting. Where do you start? You will find answering such a question much easier if you consider your response under the following headings:

- history (in this case from friends/ambulance personnel)
- examination
- special investigation
- treatment.

I will give some more examples of this type of 'what would you do next' viva question. Try to answer the question using the above scheme. The answer will be found on the following pages.

Question 1

Imagine that you are the house physician on call for the wards. It is late on Friday night and you get a call from the sister on the urology ward.

A 68–year-old man who had a transurethral prostatectomy 2 days previously has suddenly become acutely short of breath and is complaining of severe chest pains. The sister is asking you to help with his management. Your senior house officer will not be able to help you for at least 30 minutes as she has been called away to a cardiac arrest at the other side of the hospital. How would you handle this situation?

Answer

The likely causes of this patient's problem are a pulmonary embolus, myocardial infarction or a chest infection, all of which are more common in the postoperative period. Remember to think about the history, examination, special investigations and treatment with this differential diagnosis in mind.

History

The speed of onset of symptoms is an important area to cover. Symptoms from a chest infection usually come on over several hours or days. This contrasts to MI or PE where the onset is abrupt.

The type of pain may also give you a clue. In PE and chest infection the pain tends to be pleuritic, whereas in MI the pain will be typically cardiac.

You also need to ask about other possible associated symptoms, such as unilateral leg swelling (PE), haemoptysis (PE and chest infection), cough and sputum production (purulent sputum in chest infection). Asking about the past medical history may also give vital information. For example, the patient may have had a pulmonary embolus 6 months previously and has only just come off anticoagulants.

Examination

A full, thorough clinical examination is required. Mention that you will be looking for clinical signs which would help you to differentiate between the possible causes:

- chest infection
  — temperature (febrile)
  — sinus tachycardia
  — tachypnoea

— cyanosis
— unilateral signs in chest (e.g. crackles, bronchial breathing, pleural rub)
— sputum pot
- pulmonary embolus
  — sinus tachycardia
  — tachypnoea
  — central cyanosis
  — unilateral signs in chest (rub)
  — signs of DVT
- myocardial infarction
  — sweatiness, pallor
  — third heart sound/murmurs
  — bilateral inspiratory crackles (pulmonary oedema).

Investigations

Mention to the examiner that, by now, it would be likely that you would have a pretty good idea of what was wrong with the patient, but you would like some evidence to support your clinical diagnosis. This would include the following emergency investigations:

- ECG
  — ST elevation in MI
  — changes seen in PE (p. 189).
- CXR
  — pulmonary oedema (MI)
  — wedge-shaped defect in lung fields ⎫ PE
  — linear atelectasis ⎭
  — patchy unilateral signs (infection).
- FBC — The WBC is often (but not invariably) above 15 000 in a chest infection. This can sometimes help to differentiate between a PE and a chest infection when there is doubt.
- Blood gases.

Treatment

This would, of course, depend on the underlying cause.
  Chest infection.   The following should be used:

- analgesia
- O_2

- physiotherapy
- IV antibiotics.

Remember to mention that you would take blood and sputum cultures before starting the antibiotics.

Myocardial infarction/pulmonary embolus. This is rather more complicated. If the patient has had an MI he should be considered for thrombolytic therapy. If he has had a PE then intravenous heparin should be considered. However, given the fact that he has had recent surgery this may cause problems with bleeding, particularly with thrombolytic therapy. I think the correct answer is therefore:

1. analgesia
2. O_2
3. oral aspirin
4. treat pulmonary oedema (diuretic) if present.
5. seek senior advice.

Question 2

You are called to the medical admissions unit in the emergency department by a nurse. A 32-year-old woman has arrived who has quite severe dyspnoea and the nurse is worried about her. The patient's husband tells you that she was reasonably well until 40 minutes ago, when this attack started quite suddenly. He also tells you that the patient has had quite bad asthma since childhood and over the last 3 years it has been rather worse. How would you assess the severity of this patient's asthma and how would you manage her?

Answer

Again you ought to consider the history, examination, special investigations and treatment.

History

This may be difficult to obtain from the patient. If the patient is so breathless as to be unable to speak in sentences, that patient will have severe asthma. The past history is important — ask about the pattern of past attacks (e.g. history of requiring mechanical ventilation, speed of onset of symptoms, number of hospital admissions, etc.).

Examination

Assessing the severity of acute severe asthma is sometimes quite difficult. It is most important to determine whether the patient's asthma falls into the mild, moderate or severe category: it will influence your management greatly. The parameters you should look for which indicate that the patient has acute severe asthma are:

- Sinus tachycardia greater than 100 beats per minute.
- Inability to speak in sentences.
- Cyanosis.
- Pulsus paradoxus (greater than 20 mmHg).
- Silent chest (the asthma is so severe the patient is unable to get enough air in and out of the chest to create a wheeze).
- Peak flow. This needs to be related to the patient's normal measurement. A peak flow of 100 in a patient with a normal peak flow of 600 indicates very severe asthma. On the other hand, someone with a normal peak flow of 150 (who suffers with chronic asthma) who has a peak flow of 100 may only have a mild or moderate attack.

Investigations

Blood gases are an essential investigation; a falling Po_2 and a rising Pco_2 indicate that the patient is beginning to lose the battle and will require assisted ventilation. A chest X-ray is mandatory to exclude a pneumothorax, which occasionally occurs in severe asthma.

Treatment

In the treatment section you should include the use of 100% oxygen, regular nebulised bronchodilators, physiotherapy, intravenous corticosteroids, intravenous antibiotics (if indicated), intravenous aminophylline (omit the loading dose if the patient is already on theophylline derivatives), monitoring of the patient with an ECG monitor and serum theophylline levels. Patients with very severe asthma who are unresponsive to the above treatment and deteriorating may well need ventilation.

Question 3

An 18-year-old woman is brought to the Accident and Emergency department by ambulance. She was found in a semi-stuporous state by a friend with a half-empty bottle of paracetamol by her bed. What would you do next?

Answer

History

It is important to establish two facts as soon as possible. Firstly, whether the patient has taken an overdose and what tablets have been taken. Secondly, the timing of the overdose. You may need to question relatives, friends, psychiatric workers and ambulance personnel, as well as the patient. Another vital piece of information, particularly in a patient who has taken a paracetamol overdose, is an accurate alcohol and drug history. The reason for this is that chronic alcohol ingestion and the chronic use of anti-epileptics in patients who have taken a paracetamol overdose will drastically alter the threshold at which therapy with N-acetylcysteine should start.

Examination

The patient is likely to be tearful, but the rest of the examination may be normal. If she is drowsy this could imply that a large quantity of alcohol has been taken or that other tablets such as hypnotics have been taken in addition to the paracetamol.

Special investigations

These include:

- baseline clotting studies
- baseline LFT's
- serum paracetamol level.

You should mention that you would make a note of the time the paracetamol levels were taken, in relationship to the estimated time of the overdose.

Treatment

To some extent the immediate treatment depends on the quantity and timing of the paracetamol overdose. In patients who have taken only a few tablets with negligible serum paracetamol levels it is probably safe not to actively intervene. However, such patients are in the minority.

For more serious overdoses, and where there is any doubt about dose or timing, the patient should be treated with gastric lavage and be given activated charcoal orally whilst serum paracetamol levels are awaited. Once the paracetamol levels are known, a decision can be made about treatment with N-acetylcysteine. This decision is made with the help of a nomogram (see Fig. 4.1) which has serum

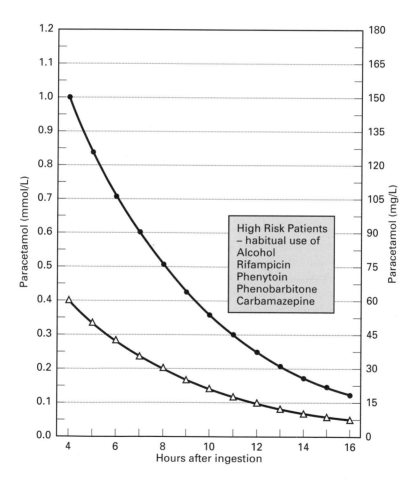

Fig. 4.1

paracetamol on the y-axis and time on the x-axis. There are several points to bear in mind about this nomogram:

1. There are two treatment lines and they are significantly different. It is vital that you categorise your patient into either the 'high risk' or 'low risk' group. If you are in any doubt categorise them as high risk.
2. Factors which will put the patient in the 'high risk' group, and therefore lower the threshold for treatment, include:
   • chronic ingestion of alcohol
   • chronic use of anti-epileptics
   • chronic use of rifampicin.
3. Serum paracetamol levels are unreliable until 4 hours have elapsed since ingestion.
4. If the patient is ANYWHERE NEAR the treatment line they should be treated. This is because there is often a certain amount of doubt about the timing of the overdose.
5. If the patient has taken a very significant amount of paracetamol, it would be reasonable to start treatment with intravenous N-acetylcysteine whilst awaiting the serum paracetamol levels.

It used to be said that N-acetylcysteine was of no use after 16 hours post-overdose. There is some evidence to suggest that this may not be the case. Furthermore, in patients who have taken a very large amount of paracetamol and the INR deteriorates, the N-acetylcysteine should be kept going. This seems to improve prognosis in patients who go on to develop acute liver failure, possibly by increasing oxygen delivery to the tissues. Clearly, a regional liver centre should be contacted about such patients.

Other aspects which should be mentioned include making contact with the regional poisons unit for expert advice, and psychiatric evaluation once the patient has finished the medical therapy.

N-acetylcysteine can cause bronchospasm, and so you should mention that special care should be taken if the patient is also asthmatic.

Other types of viva question

Occasionally examiners may ask questions relating to articles which have been in the popular press or medical journals. It is worthwhile having a look through recent copies of the *BMJ* and *Lancet* prior to your viva. Keep an eye out for medical articles in the newspapers and on TV.

Some examiners take great pleasure in asking obtuse, difficult or vague questions. Examples of such questions include:

- Tell me about the 'zoonoses' and their relationship to the Channel Tunnel.
- What are the implications of the Government's recent White Paper for the secondary care sector?
- What advice would you give a 45-year-old woman who is thinking about buying a 'home cholesterol testing kit' from the local chemist?
- What are the occupational hazards of being a postman?
- HIV is not the cause of AIDS. Discuss.

It is difficult to know what advice to give you to answer this type of mean question. However, you can take some comfort from being presented with such a question — you may well be a distinction candidate.

In summary, in the viva you need to show the examiners that you have common sense and an adequate range of medical knowledge. They will be trying to find out if you have spent any time in the Accident and Emergency department and seen treatment of emergency cases. They will also try to find out that you are up to date with current medical thinking. If you know nothing about a subject on which they are asking you questions you should tell the examiner this. More than likely he will move onto something else. Remember that they are trying to pass rather than fail you.

KEY QUESTIONS

THE VIVA VOCE

The questions below are samples of viva voce questions which students have been asked in the past.

1. **What advice would you give a 55-year-old male who had an uncomplicated myocardial infarction 10 days ago?**
2. **What is the natural history of aortic stenosis?**
3. **What is the treatment of tension pneumothorax?**
4. **How would you treat an asymptomatic 80-year-old female with blood pressure of 170/110?**
5. **What antibiotic therapy would you start (before microbiological confirmation is available) for a fit 25-year-old male with a primary community-acquired chest infection?**
6. **How would you manage a 68-year-old woman with an upper gastrointestinal haemorrhage?**
7. **What are the non-pharmacological means of therapy and support which are available for patients with HIV-associated disease? How could these be improved?**[†]
8. **What is a Sengstaken tube?**
9. **Define anaemia.**
10. **How would you assess the control of a diabetic in out-patients?**
11. **How would you manage a 40-year-old female with bloody diarrhoea?**
12. **How would you manage an 18-year-old female patient who is deeply unconscious in the casualty department?**
13. **A man falls down in front of you in the bus queue. He has no pulse and is not breathing. Describe the next 10 minutes in detail.**
14. **What are the medical risks of the combined oral contraceptive?**
15. **What is a macule? Name some conditions in which they are found.**
16. **Who was Dupuytren? What is the significance of his sign?**

Index